Injecting Bodies in More-than-Human Worlds

Drug use is widely understood in terms of its subjects, substances and settings. But what happens when these distinctions start to blur?

Injecting Bodies in More-than-Human Worlds moves away from a hierarchical conceptualisation of drug use based on its subjects and their objects, offering unique and fresh insights into the complex world of injecting drugs. Focussing on the Deleuzian notion of bodies-in-process, Dennis proposes a new and timely approach to drugs where agency materialises in relation to others – human and not. Using rich, ethnographic data to demonstrate bodies' in/capacities to act through their relationality, Dennis carefully maps out where bodies are thought, practised, lived and intervened-with: caught in tension between pleasure and addiction, activity and passivity, 'becoming-other' and 'becoming-blocked', and making and breaking habits.

Arguing for a deeper engagement both with how bodies are enacted and with our collective responsibility to bring them together in healthier ways, this volume offers a unique intervention into the sociology of drugs and, more widely, health and illness. It will appeal to students and researchers interested in fields such as Science and Technology Studies, Sociology and Social Policy, Drugs and Addiction, and Health and Medical Anthropology.

Fay Dennis is a Wellcome Trust Research Fellow in Social Science and Bioethics in the Department of Sociology at Goldsmiths, University of London.

Routledge Studies in the Sociology of Health and Illness

Fathering Children with Autism
Needs, Practices and Service Use
Carol Potter

Recovery, Mental Health and Inequality
Chinese Ethnic Minorities as Mental Health Service Users
Lynn Tang

Fertility, Health and Lone Parenting
European Contexts
Edited by Fabienne Portier-Le Cocq

Transnationalising Reproduction
Third Party Conception in a Globalised World
Edited by Róisín Ryan Flood and Jenny Gunnarsson Payne

Public Health, Personal Health and Pills
Drug entanglements and pharmaceuticalised governance
Kevin Dew

Dementia as Social Experience
Valuing Life and Care
Edited by Gaynor Macdonald and Jane Mears

Injecting Bodies in More-than-Human Worlds
Fay Dennis

For more information about this series, please visit: https://www.routledge.com/Routledge-Studies-in-the-Sociology-of-Health-and-Illness/book-series/RSSHI

Injecting Bodies in More-than-Human Worlds

Fay Dennis

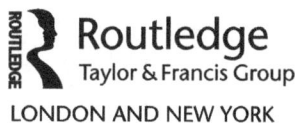

Routledge
Taylor & Francis Group

LONDON AND NEW YORK

First published 2019 by Routledge

2 Park Square, Milton Park, Abingdon, Oxfordshire OX14 4RN
52 Vanderbilt Avenue, New York, NY 10017

Routledge is an imprint of the Taylor & Francis Group, an informa business

First issued in paperback 2020

British Library Cataloguing-in-Publication Data
A catalogue record for this book is available from the British
Library

Library of Congress Cataloging-in-Publication Data
A catalog record for this book has been requested

ISBN: 978-1-138-60955-6 (hbk)
ISBN: 978-0-367-66040-6 (pbk)

Typeset in Times New Roman
by codeMantra

Rob, for too many reasons, this book is for you.

Contents

Acknowledgements

There is no book without research, and no research project without participants. Therefore, first and foremost, I would like to wholeheartedly thank everyone who took the time and emotional energy to participate in the project. I have been blown away by your generosity and willingness to share your stories with me, in many cases, a complete stranger. I only hope I have done them some justice here. I am especially thankful to those participants who went above and beyond to tell friends and peers about the study. When I was struggling to recruit women, no doubt linked to the gendered politics of drug use and under-representation of women in drug services, Lucy spread the word through her networks and I instantly started receiving calls. Because of Lucy, I was able to speak to women who were not receiving services, and this provided valuable and unique insights into these issues. I am also hugely grateful to the two service managers who allowed me to recruit from and interview people in their services. And to all the workers at the Dunswell service, where I volunteered and observed, for their daily conversations, assistance and warmth.

The research presented in this book was undertaken as part of a PhD programme at the London School of Hygiene and Tropical Medicine. I would like to thank my supervisors, Magdalena Harris and Tim Rhodes, for their support throughout this time and beyond. Magdalena used to talk about 'the book' before I could even imagine it; she planted the seed that has finally come to fruition. For their contributions and advice in the early stages of the project, I would like to acknowledge: Judy Green, Nicki Thorogood, Ford Hickson and Cicely Marston. Particular mention must be saved for Ruth Lewis who suggested I use the body mapping method, which has proven so central to the project. I am thankful to Suzanne Fraser and David Moore who hosted me at the National Drug Research Institute in Melbourne during my writing-up year. I am very grateful too to the Economic and Social Research Council whose financial support opened doctoral studies up to me.

As this research was conducted a few years ago now, there are plenty more people who have supported me through the book's production. I would like to thank the Goldsmiths Sociology Department and my new colleagues, especially Marsha Rosengarten, for welcoming me and supporting my post-doctoral fellowship. I am incredibly thankful again to Marsha and Beckie Coleman for mentoring my new research fellowship. And I am grateful to the Foundation for the Sociology of Health and Illness and the Wellcome Trust, respectively, for funding these invaluable schemes, which allowed me the time to develop the book in an otherwise challenging environment for early career academics.

I have been lucky to have the support and friendship of many colleagues: Emily Jay Nicholls, Juliet Henderson, Landon Kuester, Lucy Cullen, Polly Radcliffe, Sara Cooper and Udita Iyengar. For being there from the beginning, thank you to Emily Ross. And for being there through it all, Emma Garnett. I have been particularly touched by the collegiality and conviviality of Renae Fomiatti and Adrian Farrugia, who spent many hours reading and editing a rather disorganised and dense concluding chapter. Of course, beyond the academy, I am indebted to my friends and family that keep me grounded and joyful, you all know who you are.

I am very thankful to the four anonymous reviewers for their feedback on early drafts. They helped me sharpen the book's conceptual intervention with, hopefully, more consistency and accessibility. Thanks also to the production team at Routledge and the series editors, and to Mark Edmondson at Goldsmiths for editing the images.

This book would not be what it is without the work of many wonderful critical drug studies scholars, some of whom I have been privileged to meet and listen to at the biennial Contemporary Drug Problems conferences: Cameron Duff, Darin Weinberg, David Moore, Helen Keane, Kane Race, Kari Lancaster, Kiran Pienaar, Nicole Vitellone, Peta Malins and Suzanne Fraser.

Some of the analysis in the book reworks previously published material, including figures. I am very grateful to the publishers for their permissions to re-produce it here.

Chapter 2: Dennis, F. (2017) Conceiving of addiction pleasure: a 'modern' Paradox. *International Journal of Drug policy* 49: 150–9. (Special Issue on 'Drugged pleasures', edited by Fay Dennis and Adrian Farrugia). Published by Elsevier.

Chapters 3–4: Dennis, F. (2017) The injecting 'event': harm reduction beyond the human. Critical Public Health 27: 337–349. (Special Issue on 'Post-humanism and public health', edited by Simon Cohn and Rebecca Lynch). Published by Taylor & Francis.

Chapter 4: Dennis, F. (2016) Drugs: bodies becoming normal. M/C Journal 19(1): 1–3. (Special Issue on 'Corporeal: exploring the material dynamics of embodied', edited by Anna Lavis and Karen Eli). Published by M/C Journal – *A Journal of Media and Culture*.

Chapter 5: Dennis, F. (2016) Encountering 'triggers': drug-body-world entanglements of injecting drug use. Contemporary Drug Problems 43(2): 126–141. (Special Issue on 'Encountering alcohol and other drugs', edited by David Moore). Published by SAGE.

I want to end my acknowledgements by going back to where this book's unlikely journey started. For this, I would like to thank Long Road Sixth Form College, where for the first time I started to enjoy learning, and in particular, Karen Legge, my sociology teacher, who introduced me to the wonders of sociological thought and imagining. During my undergraduate degree, at the University of Edinburgh, I had a brilliant mentor and dissertation supervisor, Beckie Marsland, who taught me that it was okay to be critical, and in Angus Bancroft's thrilling module, Sociology of Intoxication, I learnt that I could legitimately and intellectually *do* drugs. Without these people's enthusiasm for their fields, but most importantly, their belief and encouragement, this book and my current location in a university with the time and resources to write such things would never have been possible.

Introduction
Doing drug research in more-than-human worlds

> There is a discourse on drugs current today that does no more than
> dredge up generalities on *pleasure and misfortune*, on difficulties in com-
> munication, on causes that always come from somewhere else. The more
> incapable people are of grasping a specific causality in extension, the
> more they pretend to understand the phenomenon in question.
>
> Gilles Deleuze and Félix Guattari, 1987: 283

This statement, taken from Gilles Deleuze and Félix Guattari's *A Thousand Plateaus*, first published in 1987, remains pertinent to the ways that
drug use continues to be reported, understood and treated today. Starting
to write this book, I found myself drawn towards current news stories on
drugs. Drugs have been in the news a lot recently. They are said to be killing
more people than ever in many parts of the world, including the UK, the US,
Canada and Australia. Louis Theroux's *Dark States: Heroin Town* had just
aired on British television telling the story of this epidemic in the US when I
came across a review of this programme in *The Guardian* (Wollaston, 2017).
And, there they were, the generalities, in black and white, just as Deleuze
and Guattari warned us over thirty years ago. The review painted these
'tragic' and 'bleak as hell' lives in juxtaposition with another programme
broadcast that week *Snowfall*, where the drug-taking, according to the reviewer, looked 'better; more fun, certainly'. This may seem surprising given
that it was about the 1980s US cocaine trade, with its endemic brutality
along racist, sexist and classist lines. Inadvertently highlighting how these
complex stories get reduced and reproduced, the generalities almost carica-
ture themselves. The reviewer pities the 'sad junkie lives' in *Heroin Town*, ab-
jectly describing a man's injecting site as a scab (which the presenter, Louis
Theroux, was visibly and audibly disgusted by), whilst envying the partying
lifestyles in *Snowfall*, and by contrast showing a great deal of excitement
towards a partygoer's route of cocaine administration ('up his bum'). I bring
this review to the reader's attention simply to show how readily these generalities of pleasure and misfortune circulate even amongst the so-called

liberal, left-leaning press. A series of binaries proliferate in drug reporting, researching, treatment and policymaking, which continue to make it difficult to *know* different kinds of experiences and embodiments. This book tries to tell these other stories, to do justice to the complex entanglements of bodies, drugs and worlds I encountered whilst carrying out fieldwork with people who inject drugs in these increasingly deadly times.

To return briefly to this review of *Heroin Town*, the reviewer takes an interest in one of the interviewees, Nate, who is insistent on his 'comfort' with heroin and being a 'heroin user'. But rather than exploring how this unsettles dominant narratives, this particular embodiment is forced back into line – indeed, the reviewer is quick to admire how Louis Theroux was able to unearth his comfort as 'superficial' – and thus turn Nate into just another 'tragic character' in this story of abject suffering and despair. These re-narrativisation practices resonate with my fieldwork. For example, whilst assessing a woman for treatment in my voluntary capacity as a key-worker in a drug service in London, UK, she told me how she used drugs for 'fun', and started injecting because it was something she had always wanted to try. However, giving such a reason (of pleasure, experimentation, sensation-seeking) meant she could not be ready for change and thus had to re-narrate her reasons under the guidance of a senior worker who sat beside me, towards a miscarriage she had suffered a few years prior to first injecting. It was thought that without accepting these 'real reasons', she could not be ready for change, and may instead be planning to use her opiate substitute for illicit, perhaps even pleasurable, purposes. I do not mention this story as a criticism but a way into some of the ways people's experiences get omitted by our dominant narratives on drugs. Therefore, I do not seek to address Nate's 'comfort' or this woman's 'fun' uncritically, but in fact to take these embodiments more seriously: not to be simply driven by generalities, to force them into 'misfortune', but to follow the multitude of affects, forces, experiences and embodiments that people report in their drug-taking and what this can tell us about drug use and the bodies it opens up. Rooted in ethnographic research with people who inject drugs and the people who work with them, this book seeks to get to know these otherwise silenced modes of doing drugs and the social and material processes involved.

Noticing how drug use stories are frequently re-narrativised away from pleasure, I am keen to ask difficult questions and follow alternative affects and embodied experiences. This has led to an approach to drug use based on bodies as drug-body-world relations and the ways we mediate these relations in producing drug 'effects' – embodiments and experiences. I say 'we' because as our bodies get broken down beyond these biological boundaries, we all become involved in the ways bodies are made, and thus, how they can be made better. This builds on a growing field of critical drug studies explicitly engaged with theories that disrupt the human subject or individual traditionally positioned at the heart of drug studies and sociology more generally. Drawing on thought from new materialisms, science and technology studies, and process philosophy, researchers and commentators show how 'drug effects' are contingent on the coming together of various networks or assemblages of human and non-human processes in more-than-human worlds.

This book builds on these traditions, paying attention to three trends in particular. That is, where, in our more-than-human worlds, the primary unit of analysis shifts, according to Cameron Duff (2017), from the drug-using subject to 'the event', drug 'effects' are no longer dependent on the *choices of the user*, the *essence of the substance* or even *the context*, be it material or discursive. Drawing from the philosophy of Gilles Deleuze, the drug event is contingent on a complex interaction of these bodies, technologies and forces, where one does not precede or exist outside of the other. I will next look at how these disruptions have occurred: first, to 'the human', second, to 'the substance' and, third, to 'the context'. This will carve the way for a new kind of drug study, one that is sensitive to the emergent, processual and contingent nature of drug-taking and -treatment events and their embodiments.

Disrupting 'the human'

The decision-making, rational individual has proven to be an important figure for both sociological and public health understandings of drug use. A prominent line of argument in sociology has been to rationalise otherwise, in accordance with our dominant ideals of rationality, irrational practices of intoxication. Sociology has worked tirelessly to find meaning where there is seemingly none. In one of the earliest sociological accounts of British drug taking, Jock Young (1971) looked at the 'social meaning of heroin use', namely, for escaping the tedium and alienation of capitalist modes of production, with its false promises of joy from mass consumption. Howard Becker (1953) in the US famously explored how marijuana was reinterpreted as enjoyable through one's social relationships and meaning-making. Following these early traditions, sociological studies have focussed on understanding drug users as rational subjects, who meaningfully navigate late-modern landscapes, often as an antidote to alarmist media coverage, 'just say no' education-programmes, punitive legal frames and pathologising medical narratives. In *Illegal Leisure,* a seminal work of the 1990s in the sociology of drug use, Howard Parker, Judith Aldridge and Fiona Measham (1998) highlight the 'rational cost/benefit analysis' at the heart of adolescent drug taking for achieving a 'time-out' from the 'uncertain and "risky" post-modern world' (1998: 2). Known as the 'normalisation thesis', drug use is seen as a 'normal' practice of postmodern society.[1]

Professor of Criminology at Durham University, UK, Fiona Measham has been a particularly important voice in this rationalisation movement in Britain – working to rationalise people's decisions to take drugs and the ways they are taken. Her work on gender (2000; 2002) and leisure spaces (2004) in the nightclub and rave scene demonstrated how drug use was part of what she coined a 'controlled loss of control' – a controlled 'form of escape' from the 'surveillance and regulation of consumer society' (2004: 344). 'The "controlled loss of control" is a calculated hedonistic act which aims to achieve a desired, structured and controllable altered state of intoxication, by pharmacological or behavioural intervention' (Measham, 2004: 343). In highlighting the intentionality behind intoxication, a number of similar terms have evolved to rationalise alcohol and other drug (AOD)-using experiences.

'Determined drunkenness' is employed to emphasise the thought-processes in an otherwise seemingly accidental practice (Hutton, 2012; Measham, 2006). 'Calculated hedonism' (Brain, 2000; Featherstone, 1991; Fry, 2011) accounts for 'a type of pleasure which is contained by time, space and social situation' (Szmigin et al., 2008: 365): 'there is a dimension to their consumption of control; this may not be apparent to onlookers at the times when the young people are drinking excessively but *they are choosing* when, where and who to drink with' (2008: 362, my emphasis). 'Bounded consumption' (Szmigin et al., 2008) and 'bounded loss of control' (Measham and Brain, 2005) similarly denote the way people use AODs within individually and/or socially set 'bounds'. Moreover, 'staged intoxication' is used to capture how intoxication is 'staged', where 'pleasure is only achieved if the *right* drink is drunk in the *right* context, at the *right* time' (Lindsay, 2009: 376, my emphasis).

Where sociological approaches to AODs have reordered 'recreational' drug use as both individually controlled and socially meaningful, from a similar position, a 'social science *for* harm reduction' (Rhodes, 2009) emerged during this period with perhaps an even tougher task of giving meaning to practices of drug use that are deemed dependent or addictive. Harm reduction is a public health approach to drug use based on 'policies, programmes and practices that aim primarily to reduce the adverse health, social and economic consequences of the use of legal and illegal psychoactive drugs without necessarily reducing drug consumption' (IHRA, 2010: 1). In this area of public health, social researchers reveal why and how people consume drugs and the reasons for their chosen routes of administration to inform policies and practices to reduce the risk of harm.

A central tenant of the harm reduction movement in the UK, as a response to the human immunodeficiency virus (HIV) in the 1990s (MacGregor, 2017; Stimson, 2007), was to position drug users as rational citizens, who, given the correct information, technologies and facilities, will make informed choices to reduce drug-related harm. Fearful that people who inject drugs would act as conduits for HIV, taking the virus into the general population, notoriously conservative policymakers were forced to support previously unacceptable programmes, such as needle exchanges. To make this leap, as Virginia Berridge points out in her extensive writing on the area, 'a potentially controversial policy shift [to the principles of harm reduction away from a previous focus on abstention] was transferred into the realm of "science" through the medium of research and evaluation' (1999: 37). This 'transition' is highlighted in the very first International Conference on the Reduction of Drug Related Harm held in Liverpool, UK, in 1990, which called for drug policy with less moralism and more *rationalism* (O'Hare et al., 1992), and again it is seen in the third Conference, aptly entitled 'Psychoactive Drugs and Harm Reduction: *From Faith to Science*' (Heather et al., 1993, my emphasis). By neutralising these harm reduction programmes as scientific and 'evidence-based' (Berridge, 1999), people who use drugs were rationalised as capable of engaging in such technologies. The 'irrational drug user', or worse, 'junkie', concerned only with getting high or self-destructing, became a citizen-patient, capable of self-care (Drumm et al., 2005; Gowan et al., 2012; Roe, 2005). Seen now as somebody equally interested in health, 'the drug user' became helpable and advocates of harm reduction seized on this opportunity to develop more compassionate and effective interventions (Erickson et al., 1997; Reinarman and Levine, 1997).

However, this model of harm reduction relies on people privileging health. What happens if/when people who use drugs fail to choose health? Or, as the famous opening scene of the internationally acclaimed British film of this era, *Trainspotting*, goes, choose not to 'choose life', but choose something else, like, as we have seen above, pleasure, intimacy or comfort? Or, even, whether, by showing the constrained and often oppressive conditions of these 'choices', what happens if these people's practices challenge the very notion and limits of choice and freedom? Therefore, around this time, a critical harm reduction narrative also emerged to understand these 'alternative rationalities'. That is, where health professionals were seen to view 'informed choices to act riskily or dangerously [as] irrational', a critical harm reduction movement took a 'situated' approach (Rhodes, 1997).[2] Arguing against what he calls a 'single rationality', Tim Rhodes (1995; 1997; 2009), in developing a 'social science *for* harm reduction', makes the case for drug policies and interventions to take account of a 'situated rationality', where decisions are taken in specific social and economic environments (see also Bourgois, 1998; Moore, 2004; Rhodes and Hartnoll, 1996; Rhodes et al., 2003).

Injecting, for example, as a route of drug administration, which is linked to a heightened risk of blood borne virus transmission and therefore, in a public health setting, is mostly seen as devoid of rationality, as an outcome of desperation and necessity, is challenged by social scientists in search for alternative or what are sometimes called 'indigenous' forms of rationality (Harris and Rhodes, 2013a). Critical drug scholars have found a myriad of reasons for why people may choose to inject rather than smoke heroin, including its cost-effectiveness, discreteness, share-ability, and capacity to engender pleasure, intimacy and closeness to one's injecting partner (e.g. Bravo et al., 2003; Fraser, 2013; Giddings et al., 2003; Harris and Rhodes, 2012; Ivsins and Marsh, 2018; Rhodes et al., 2017; Vitellone, 2003a; Witteveen et al., 2006). Like the sociological literature on recreational drug use, these scholars seek to identify reason, meaning and control where, dictated by dominant discourses of what rationality looks like (based on individual freedom and control), there is seemingly none.

In a similar way to the 'recreational drug user', the 'situated' harm reduction figure retains some of the rational features of the neoliberal subject it seeks to critique. A strategic use of the neoliberal subject or individual is not only reflexively challenged by critical drug researchers, but also often endorsed as necessary (Moore and Fraser, 2006). During the 1990s, a number of studies, influenced by the work of Michel Foucault, and especially his concepts of governmentality and biopower, started to criticise the potential disciplining effects of harm reduction and warned its sympathisers that they could be perpetuating rather than challenging the structures that pathologise and oppress people who use drugs (e.g. Bergschmidt, 2004; Bourgois, 2000; Mclean, 2011; Moore, 2004; Roe, 2005). Indeed, as early as the third International Conference on the Reduction of Drug Related Harm, Mugford questioned the 'naivety of "liberation"' and 'limits of "reason"' (1993: 31). In an essay by Moore and Fraser (2006), they carefully pit the merits of using the neoliberal subject *for* harm reduction against its normalising and disciplining tendencies. Its uncritical use is problematised for constraining other ways of being *with* drugs and in treatment settings – those addicted ways of being that threaten rationality and those forms of pleasure that stigmatise its service-using subjects as 'non-conformists' for 'failing the test' of neoliberal rationalism (2006: 3045). They argue, conversely, however, that the neoliberal subject may also be the most readily available figure for improving the health outcomes of those who use drugs. Two years previously, Helen Keane also asserted how 'the recruitment of drug users into programmes of disease prevention can be negatively classified as the production of disciplined subjects, but it also enables these drug-using subjects to make new demands of authorities and claims about their needs' (2003: 231). These programmes, simply by existing and providing support, can allow for new kinds of subjectivity. Given the chance, that is, if we hold off from a quick critique of the structural inequalities and disciplining powers of these technologies, they may potentialise other, more agentic ways of being. And these may, if we are careful and diligent in our observations, expose processes of subjectivation which, unlike the neoliberal subject, are not so dependent on ideals of freedom and control.

Taking this point further, I want to look next at some of these processes of subjectivation in the drug-using and -treatment event and how these disrupt the human subject as in any way 'given' or *a priori*. More specifically, through a select few studies (which are by no means exhaustive), I wish to explore how these more-than-human processes, unlike the rational neoliberal subject above, allow for a *lack of control*, the agency of the *body* and *nonhuman materiality* as subjects emerge through the drug-using/treatment event.

Lack of control

In Darin Weinberg's (2013) essay on 'the missing core of addiction science', he criticises the natural sciences and social sciences alike for failing to recognise, theorise and intervene with a loss of control, which he sees at the heart of addiction. He writes that drug use has been seen as a 'deviant but nonetheless self-governed behaviour' (2013: 173). Using Bruno Latour's concept of the body as a 'learning faculty in its own right', he reinvigorates the notion of a loss of self-control as a set of learnt practices and embodied sensitivities, positioning addiction as a firmly embodied phenomenon (see also Weinberg, 2002). The drug is seen to reside inside the user who is losing control – 'to *inhabit* them or engage and be engaged by them' (2013: 179, original emphasis). Whilst I do not necessarily agree with this need to reinstate addiction as a loss of control, or to find its 'core', or even whether this is possible, for me, this essay does important work for fleshing out a process of subjectivation that does not have to rely on control. Subjectivation is a process that is thoroughly contingent on the sensitivity of both human and non-human components such that the substance and body adjust to one another in a dually material and agential way.

Furthering this ambition to take a lack of control seriously, but without firming up a notion of addiction, researchers have critiqued the 'controlled loss of control' thesis, arguing that drug enactments cannot be controlled by the user (Bundy and Quintero, 2017; Dennis, 2016; Poulsen, 2015). But rather than invoking a loss of control, Meret Poulsen suggests, perhaps, a shared control in which 'agency is understood to be shaped by the intra-actions that make up a phenomenon' (2015: 13). Engaging with Karen Barad's philosophy of agential realism, Poulsen traces the ways gendered and sexualised subjectivities emerge in drug encounters, namely on the dance floor. The 'control' that participants expressed over their drug practices is always in connection to others, human and non-human, stretching beyond a 'humanist notion of agency and control' (2015: 13). She shows how participant's descriptions of intoxication or 'breaking down', as one participant describes it, could not be 'managed' by the subject in the way that a 'controlled loss of control' may suggest. Rather, there are fields of possibilities, 'possibilities that cannot be possessed by an individual', where different 'parts' of the field (sociomaterially 'cut') have different capacities – 'these relations include alcohol, music, light, affectivity, other bodies, spatial "vibes," and time'

(2015: 13). Calculated hedonism (Fry, 2011), Poulsen argues, and one might also include all the other concepts discussed above that prefix an embodied experience of intoxication with a cognitive adverb, cannot answer for the forces that flow through these relations that mean although certain affects and effects may be desired, they are not necessarily realised, as participants describe scenes of 'chaos'. Hedonism, Poulsen argues, fails to account for these forces of desire that exist beyond the cognitive in our relationality, and the very pull to experiment and experience things that cannot be explained, in changing the 'field of possibilities for being' (2015: 14).

'The body'

Through both works by Weinberg and Poulsen, the body and embodiment are foregrounded in a resolutely more-than-human way, made up of human and non-human processes. This again disrupts the dominant recreational drug user and harm reduction figure as a rational decision-maker. Weinberg draws on theorists such as Donna Haraway, as well as Latour, to elide an ontological differentiation between 'the social' and 'the biological', which is seen to underpin a sociological neglect of the body and new embodiments. Latour's (2004a) notion of the body as 'learning to be affected' illuminates 'the lived realities of embodiment by revealing the body as not only the mechanical medium through which our minds learn but an intrinsically developing and learning faculty in its own right' (Weinberg, 2013: 177). The body becomes a site of thoughtfulness, reflection and ultimately agency (also see Race, 2017; 2018). By considering the agency of the body, made up within and through its context, this broadens our understanding of drug effects such as pleasure beyond the rational 'wherein the pleasurability of drug effects is not a neurological fait accompli but derives to a considerable extent from perceptions of a felicitous fit between drug effects and the practical demands of specific situations' (Weinberg, 2013: 178).

For Weinberg and Poulsen, as we have seen, there is a loss of control or shared control in these embodiments. The body is central to these processes of subjectivation, otherwise neglected by theories of the neoliberal subject. This is influenced by and extends Peta Malins' (2004; 2007; 2017) important writings on the drug-using body. Following a close reading of Gilles Deleuze, (and Félix Guattari) her work also informs the approach taken in this book (to be discussed at length in Chapter 4) as a decisively anti-individualist ethicopolitics, committed to the body as an assemblage. Her famous essay 'Machinic assemblages: Deleuze, Guattari and an ethico-aesthetics of drug use' is one of the best examples of a Deleuzo-Guattarian approach to drug use through articulations of the body (also see Fitzgerald, 1998; Fitzgerald and Threadgold, 2007; Malins, 2004; 2007; Malins et al., 2006).

In a slightly different vein, other researchers working on heroin use have similarly been drawn to the body 'to overcome the mentalist or cognitive privileging that is inherent in earlier work' (Nettleton et al., 2011: 343). A sentiment summed up in Nettleton and colleagues' paper title: 'I don't think there's much of a rational mind in a drug addict when they are in the thick of it'. Writing in relation to 'drug recovery', they argue that the literature 'has tended to focus on rational, cognitive and symbolic dimensions of action to the relative neglect of pre-reflective, non-symbolic, and crucially, embodied action' (2011: 341). Using Shilling's (2008) concept of 'habitual action' to understand the *embodied* and *relational* aspects of '[drug] using bodies', Nettleton et al. argue that recovery 'involves embodied subjects discovering *routinised* models of behaviour that are more or less effective in "joining" them to, and enabling them to manage their surroundings' (2011: 344). This is not the same as saying bodies are dependent on non-human others, but that our embodied actions of everyday life leave us always entwined with others.

Looking further at the somatic aspects of heroin injecting, this time from a phenomenological perspective, Harris, in her personal account of hepatitis C stigma and injecting, reflects on the visceral 'latent desire' that causes her body to 'contract' at the sight of a syringe (2009: 40). She highlights the embodied nature of injecting, which includes a lasting embodiment on the skin (in scars) and under the skin (in bodily memories) of 'intense highs' along with 'desperation' (2009: 36). Taken up further in a more recent article, she reflects more broadly on the bodily practices of qualitative research, honing in on her own 'heroin memories' – 'a tension between repulsion and desire that pops up in and around [her] interview practice' (Harris, 2015: 4, my emphasis). These visceral (and automatic) responses highlight the embodiment of drug use, which offers a way of going beyond the rational and bounded pleasure seeker (in the recreational drug user figure) or health-seeker (in the harm reduction figure). In disrupting the human, we disrupt human agency at the site of the mind, opening up agentic possibilities to the body, and next, non-human materiality.

Non-human materiality

To centre on human rationality and reason in drug-taking is to neglect the role of material things, objects and technologies in processes of subjectivation. Over the last five years or so, the AOD field has been experiencing a sustained shift towards 'the material' (see journal special issues by Duff, 2013; Dennis and Farrugia, 2017; Seear and Moore, 2014), which follows similar trends across the social sciences.[3] Exposing this gap and the need to address it, Duff writes:

> Ascribing a capacity for agency to substances themselves, to *material* spaces and settings, sound systems, music, fashion, shoes and mobile phones, might offend *humanist* assumptions about the character of *free will, intentionality and choice*; yet, it is critical if one hopes to

develop more nuanced accounts of the everyday experience of AOD consumption.

(Duff, 2012: 155, my emphasis)

Whilst an interest in materiality is by no means new (Gomart and Hennion, 1999), and indeed, arguably responds to a long history of the 'risk environment' (Rhodes, 2002; 2009), it has only more recently gained widespread traction.

In its current guise, it responds to a dissatisfaction with social constructionist ideas of drug use, seen to prioritise 'the social' and 'the human'. Duff's work highlights the role of the material in ontologically disrupting any notion of a rational subject existing outside/*a priori* to the drug-using event. 'Singling out one actor in this network – such as the consuming subject – without acknowledging the agency of the myriad additional actors involved in this consumption merely reinforces the quaint dogma of rational choice' (Duff, 2012: 155). Instating the drug-using *event* as the 'primary unit of analysis' and subjects, rather than existing before, emerging through these events (Duff, 2014a; 2017), the subject is recast as more-than-human.

Suzanne Fraser and kylie valentine (2008), for example, look at the ways subjects are made *with* the opiate substitute, methadone, as 'methadone subjects'. More recently, spending time in drug consumption rooms in Frankfurt, Germany, Duncan and colleagues (2017) recognise the way subjects come to be made in such spaces, and thus, the real possibilities to engender better subjectivities in their speculative design. In contrast to the public injecting spaces, marked by fear of arrest, and stigmatisation from the public, which means rushing to inject in a vein, potentialising an injury, supervised injecting clinics, through the affective flows produced by the café area, 'friendly staff' and sterile equipment are shown to (as suggested above by Keane, 2003) potentialise 'healthier' and even more joyous subjectivities. These constructions of subjects are something we must recognise in our interventions, and attempts have been made to engender the 'freedoms' (Harris and Rhodes, 2013a) and 'relationships' (Fraser et al., 2017) that harm reduction technologies are otherwise seen to constrain.

As a closing remark on how the human subject in sociological accounts of recreational drug use and public health accounts of harm reduction has been disrupted by our more-than-human worlds, these processes of drugged subjectivation should not be thought of as completely sporadic or undetermined, but rather, as Dilkes-Frayne and Duff (2017) have recently argued, a matter of continuity and change. That is, thinking with Brian Massumi, 'where continuity is an effect of an accrual of tendencies in bodies, and where change is introduced precisely at the moment at which tendencies are actualised differently' (Dilkes-Frayne and Duff, 2017: 8). Let me describe this argument briefly before concluding on where this takes a critical study of drugs to next.

Focussing on one participant's story, Dilkes-Frayne and Duff look at the tendencies involved in what he recounts as a random event of methylene-dioxymethamphetamine (MDMA) use (a friend turning up with a surprise package at the pub), and the multiple potentials actualised as the night took shape, organised around going out with his friends or, as he had previously agreed (before the 'surprise package' arrived and the substance was ingested), returning home with his partner. In the end, the course of the night took a similar one to that originally planned, the participant went home. Nonetheless, the authors diligently and creatively depict the alternative lines that were partially actualised, with no body or thing being in control, asking 'who (or what) will decide where these encounters lead?' (2017: 10). But neither are these courses completely random as subjective qualities endure and get repeated. 'Materialised in the repetitions of practice, gesture and routine, (drug-using) tendencies may become stable over time if they are actualised in similar ways in subsequent events, or dissipate if they are not' (Dilkes-Frayne and Duff, 2017: 955). Therefore, perhaps this homeward trajectory is not so surprising after all, as a tendency that is more habituated than going out. Although subjects are always in process, becoming-other, they do not start anew, but rather constantly repeat, and it is in these moments that change is possible. Reinvigorating a focus on subjectivation and subjectivities where post-human enquiry, according to Dilkes-Frayne and Duff, has tended to look at the momentary (often one-off) event, harm reduction efforts, they argue, should 're-direct the tendencies and trajectories that carry bodies – human and nonhuman – into and out of events' (2017: 14). So, not only is the event of importance, but so too are these tendencies and trajectories that inform and extend it. As such, Dilkes-Frayne and Duff point to new modes of governing or harm reduction praxis based on 'paying attention' (Gonçalves et al., 2016) and 'ethics' (Duff, 2015) as an 'alternative means for intervening' that is not dependent on the human subject (2017: 14).

In more-than-human worlds, where human subjects can no longer be isolated in the way they once were, it makes little sense to focus on drug users' meaning-making and decision-making as if they exist outside/beyond these drug-using events. This is something that drug users have been telling us all along as they so evidently, often joyously, live *with* significant non-human others. Attuning to these processes of subjectivation, decisions cannot be made in advance or outside of these events and are only known as right/wrong, good/bad within them. Therefore, to place too much emphasis on individual decision-making – Why do people use drugs? Why in these certain ways? What are the costs/benefits? How do people maximise the good/reduce the harms? – is to ask too much (Duff, 2014b), and, as we have seen, to neglect a *lack of control*, the role of *the body* and *nonhuman materiality*. Next, I turn to how these more-than-human worldings disrupt the very substance that is seen to be consumed or injected.

Disrupting 'the substance'

Substances, taken to alter or enhance moods and bodies, are a defining feature of modern society (Boothroyd, 2004; Manning, 2007). As commentators have put it, illicit substances are embedded in our 'rave new world' (Phaphides, 1997), and their consumers are merely 'medicated followers of fashion' (Collin, 1996). In the UK, this embeddedness of substances in society can be traced to the opium dens of the nineteenth century. More recent historical examples include the use of amphetamines in 1970s Northern Soul (Wilson, 2007), cannabis in reggae sound-system movements (Gilroy, 2005), ecstasy in 1990s rave scenes (Malbon, 1999; Reynold, 1999) and alcohol in the noughties 'binge drinking' culture (Measham and Brain, 2005). Substances have been both admired for their creativity and despised for their destructivity. There is perhaps no substance more controversial, that is, caught up in these tensions, than heroin (Hussey, 2014). Heroin, until the 1970s, was mostly prescribed by doctors to the London elite, but with brown, smokable heroin imported from Iran and mass deindustrialisation, it became increasingly popular from the 1980s across the UK, especially in deprived areas. With the rise of the HIV/AIDS in the late 1980s and 1990s, heroin, which was increasingly 'cooked up' into a soluble solution for injecting, became more stigmatised than ever as a potential transmitter of disease, and its creative potential once present in, for example, 1940s Jazz or 1950s beat generation literature and poetry began to overwhelmingly signify suffering and misery (Vitellone, 2015; 2017).

At the same time that illicit substances have revealed themselves to be embedded in culture (for good or bad), modern medicine and science has become just as concerned with trying to isolate substances from culture: to locate the causal effects of psychoactive drugs in the brain. This is especially the case for those drugs considered addictive (Vrecko, 2010), but also increasingly for so-called recreational drugs. *The Ecstasy Trial*, broadcast on mainstream UK television in 2012, is a telling example (Channel 4, 2012). It showed neuropsychopharmacologist, Professor David Nutt, once head of the government's Advisory Council on the Misuse of Drugs,[4] conducting a randomised control trial (RCT) into ecstasy's neurological effects. Participants were given MDMA (chemical name for ecstasy), left in a room for the drug to take effect, and then scanned using magnetic resonance imaging to localise the drug's impact in the brain. But as anybody who has taken ecstasy, or any psychoactive drug for that matter, will tell you, 'its' effects are hugely contingent on the environment in which it is taken – the music, lights, people, space, temperature, etc. Therefore, by trying to isolate ecstasy's activation in the brain within this controlled environment, the experiment not only neglects these contingent factors, but shuts down the multiple qualities and potential directions the substance can take with the body. The substance is quashed before it is given a chance to engage the participant in different ways. And, as the scientists in the trial find out, some participants felt underwhelmed and disappointed with the effects, wishing they could have had a higher dose.

However, in privileging the social and cultural aspects of drug use, the social sciences have been equally neglectful of the substance and what it has to offer. Drugs have been left largely intact as 'matters of fact'. In contrast, in her book, *What's Wrong with Addiction?*, Helen Keane destabilises the substance, explaining its multiple ontologies through Derrida's figure of the pharmakon as both poison and cure. The pharmakon notably 'cannot be fixed in oppositions of good/evil, true/false, inside/outside, but rather disrupts these terms', removing any notion that substances have essences and causal effects (Keane, 2002: 14). Considering substances like subjects, as events in themselves, offers a unique point of insight and entry into the coming together of culture, bodies and technologies. Substances, therefore, can be good cure-like medicines or bad poison-like drugs depending on their encounters with other bodies, technologies and environments (2002: 35). In this section, I focus mainly on the literature on licit drugs or medicines as work on the multiplicity of illicit substances is rare. By paying attention to these encounters, I look at the way the substances in these accounts are enacted as already *cultural, multiple, contingent* and *bodily*.

'Cultural'

In an editorial collection for the journal *Science as Culture*, Suzanne Fraser, kylie valentine and Celia Roberts (2009) explore, with their contributors, the lives of drugs as 'social and political agents' in current medicalisation practices. Taking the intriguing substance of Suboxone as their focus, which is made up of the partial opioid agonist buprenorphine and the opioid antagonist naloxone, they explore its inbuilt sociality. Used as a substitute for heroin addiction, if injected it sends the user into precipitated withdrawals. In one of the most visceral ways possible, 'particular cultures are literally folded into the materiality of certain drugs', inscribing and punishing the 'social prohibition against injecting' (2009: 125). This can also be seen in light of a corpus of work on the more usual opiate substitute, methadone, where it has been positioned as a disciplining technology, especially through its delivery (e.g. Bergschmidt, 2004; Bourgois 2000; Friedman and Alicea, 2001). Methadone recipients often have to attend clinics or pharmacies for their dose and are watched by staff to ensure the whole dose is taken. A number of issues ensue from these practices: queues can form and become crowded and tense as people wait; recipients are not only subjected to the gaze of the medical professional who watches them but in pharmacies, members of the public too; the dose, heavily controlled by the medical providers, can be felt to be too sedating or indeed not enough to stave off withdrawal symptoms; the dose has to be taken in one, and cannot be staggered as some recipients prefer; doses can be withdrawn if the recipient misses the dosing time or their appointment with the doctor to obtain a prescription; and whether the recipient is able to take their methadone home (further on in their treatment) can become a bargaining tool to end their illicit use of heroin and other drugs (Bourgois, 2000; Fraser, 2006; Fraser and valentine, 2008; Harris and Rhodes, 2013a; Keane, 2009). Methadone is both embedded in these cultural restraints and enacted through these practices. Taking this position further, however, considering shifts to 'the material', this is not simply about the medicalisation of drug use as a disciplining technique, but about the ways substances and medicines can also act and resist such discourses. Drawing from Karen Barad (2007), this is about how the world 'kicks back'. In other words, substances too help to enact themselves, gaining their capacities to act through these events in which they are only partially brought into being.

Multiple substances

In a recent review of the medicalisation of cannabis in Victoria, Australia, Kari Lancaster and colleagues (2017) show how 'medical cannabis' actively engages and disrupts existing ways of organising substances. Getting involved in these binaries of 'recreational abuse' versus 'medicinal cure', the authors look at the ways cannabis is made in policy. Rather than predating 'the problem' of medical cannabis, the substance is created in its 'problematisation' (Bacchi, 2009; 2012) – 'how "medical cannabis" relies on the "absent presence" of "recreational cannabis"'. Medical cannabis, they argue, enacts a broader sense of health and well-being which could open up discourses often foreclosed to medicine. That is, in exploring how medical cannabis is made, the authors seek to explore how it could be 'made otherwise' (Law and Singleton, 2000; Mol 1999). Extending what a medicine is and can be, medicinal cannabis disrupts the usual divisions set up between medicine/drug and therapy/recreation. This hints to where the substance can take us, not as a product of its chemical makeup (essence), or simply determined by 'the social' or 'cultural' milieu it finds itself in, but as actively creating new ways of relating, modes, in this case, that have not been possible under prohibition.

Drawing also from Bacchi's (2009) problematisation thesis ('What's the Problem Represented to be?'), Tim Rhodes (2018) conceptualises the changing nature of methadone in East Africa as always 'in becoming'. 'The becoming of methadone' incapsulates how methadone gets made and remade through its sociomaterial environment, constituting different kinds of treatment or intervention in different space-times. Recently implemented in East Africa, according to the UN, methadone is a technology of HIV prevention, but in interview accounts with methadone's users, it is presented 'as a technology of drug withdrawal alleviation, enabling addiction recovery' and promising 'normalcy' (2018: 74). Rhodes looks at 'moments of evidence-making' in hear-say and embodied knowledge. 'These moments in evidence-making are also afforded relative security and longevity since the embodiment of methadone as a good is located among former methadone doubters of the drug world' (2018: 76). Methadone is not one substance, but multiple, and its evidential qualities do not inform, but are made *through* its implementation.

To extend this point in relation to a different drug, albeit one again of HIV prevention, Michael and Rosengarten show how Pre-Exposure Prophylaxis or PrEP, 'a pill taken every day that ostensibly decreases the risk of HIV infection', is 'event-ualised', that is, how it is 'made manifest in particular events in which many entities and relations are brought together (bodies, science, ethics, health workers, pills etc.)' (2013: 9). Interested particularly in the RCT as a site of this eventuation, Michael and Rosengarten trace the multiplicity of PrEP as it is enacted in different topologies, disrupting its 'universal applicability' to be taken at any time or place (2013: 145). The evidence of PrEP, like methadone, is therefore multiply constituted as it is enacted and stabilised through these different assemblages.

Emergent causality

Following on from the above, evidence is made in the intervention rather than constituting its basis. This is what Rhodes and colleagues (2016) call 'evidence making (rather than "based") intervention'. No longer can interventions or medicines be isolated and known 'objectively', but are remade every time they are eventuated. In a similar way to the MDMA story told by Dilkes-Frayne and Duff (2017) above, which problematised subjectivity (at least fully constituted) existing prior to the consumption event, this disrupts any prior causality and invokes what Kane Race (2014) has understood through William Connolly as 'emergent causality'. In relation to the use of sniffer dogs at Sydney Gay and Lesbian Mardi Gras, Race writes that 'emergent causality makes it possible to see how any element in a given assemblage can acquire contingent agentic capacities' (2014: 301). Causalities can only come about in the event as they rely on the specific combination of the components that enter it, but also how these components register each other. Therefore, to some extent at least, the 'components' of the event bring each other into being and cannot exist beforehand. Race calls for more sensitivity in registering these emergent causalities in how, in his case, police dogs enable and/or disable certain drug practices and bodies. One trajectory he observes and is concerned by is how police dogs may work to deter people from going out to clubs and bars, leading to an increased use of online hook-ups and socialising in private homes. As forms of sociality change, moving to the virtual and private sphere, a new set of outcomes are potentialised as people may not be able to access the help they need if at risk of overdose or sexual assault. But equally pressing for Race, segregated forms of sociability and sexuality may foreclose productive and not-yet-imaginable modes of public expression, engagement and politics (2014, see also 2017; 2018).

Substance-bodies

If substances come into being through their specific constructing events – be it in their consumption, or for Rhodes, and Michael and Rosengarten, in 'the intervention', or for Lancaster and colleagues, in policymaking – they, to a certain extent, make themselves known in their coming-into-being with other human and non-human bodies. So, far from predicting or evidencing, we can only ever speculate on their effects. For Michael and Rosengarten, thinking with Alfred North Whitehead, medicines are 'always eventuated in their specificity' (2012: 7). 'Accordingly, the body and medicine do not exist in the abstract – as primary qualities to which secondary qualities are attached' (2012: 7). To quote from the epigraph, drugs do not exist 'in extension'. Drawing on 'inventive problem making' (Fraser, 2010), rather than say problematisation (in both Foucault's and Bacchi's rendering), this is about putting into 'dialogue the "abstraction of practice" and "practice of abstraction"' (Michael and Rosengarten, 2012: 14). Michael and Rosengarten (2012) therefore ask: What kinds of abstraction do drug practices make possible? Like substances do not simply exist within a culture but produce culture, substances are not only consumed or utilised by bodies, but also *do* bodies. Notably, substances are not solely controlling mechanisms, embroiled in wider social structures, as methadone is frequently seen (Bergschmidt, 2004; Bourgois, 2000), but entities that can resist and make themselves known in new and different ways. For example, as pleasurable *and* curative in the case of cannabis, as new kinds of recovery potential in the case of methadone, or as 'medium', 'product' and 'affect' in the case of PrEP.

To conclude this section on disrupting the substance, far from substances existing outside culture, or outside the body, in a way that is predictable and measurable, they materialise at points of curious eventuation of diverse and seemingly unconnected practices, forces and technologies. Culture is enmeshed in the substance as much as substances have always been enmeshed in culture. To separate these out in any clear way is merely superficial and could at once give too much power, and with it responsibility, to the *consumer* as 'master' of the substance, the *substance* as 'master' (at least pharmacologically) of the consumer, or even *culture* as an overriding dictator of it all (as in social constructionism). Instead, we need to consider the intimate interaction or 'intra-action' (as Karen Barad says) of human and non-human processes as already entangled in substance-making. Following these arguments, a critical study of drug use is further complicated by a disruption to 'the context'.

Disrupting 'the context'

> 'Context' is one of the most enduring analytical devises in social science accounts of alcohol and other drug use.
>
> Cameron Duff, 2014b: 633

In contrast to the 'natural sciences' that try to localise drug effects, most recently in the brain, which dominates how we understand and notably fund addiction studies,[5] the cultural, structural and discursive contexts of drug use have been central to social scientists' understandings of how and why people take drugs. For Jock Young, 'the task, therefore, is to explain the origins and content of the *culture* the drug-taker belongs to and then, and only then, the role drugs play in it' (1971: 60, my emphasis). Howard Becker's (1953) classic work on learning to be a marijuana smoker, which informs Young's approach, is similarly dependent on the cultural appropriation of technique, feelings and ultimately enjoyment from 'the group'. And Norman Zinberg's (1984) study in the 1980s builds on these traditions in cementing sociological interest in the 'setting' as central to how drugs come to have their effect, and the meanings people find in their experiences. In recent years, however, as our more-than-human worlds have made themselves known, this focus on the context has come under fire for privileging the human, both in prioritising the social in social contexts and positioning the human at the centre of contexts, more generally, as the organising, 'situated' and 'situating' agent.

Following this shift to 'the material' (noted above), contexts are no longer seen in terms of positioning human subjects, their choices to consume what, where and how, but *with* subjects, *as* assemblages, networks or entanglements. Dissatisfied with both structural and social constructionist ideas of drug use, which are seen to continue to prioritise 'the social' and 'the human', researchers have been drawn to theories that flatten out these relationships between subjects and objects in following their attachments (e.g. Demant, 2009; Dilkes-Frayne, 2014; Gomart and Hennion, 1999). Considering again the experience of pleasure, researchers have explored how rather than pleasure being 'chosen' by a subject and sanctioned socially by the group or wider discourses of advanced liberalism (in risk-taking and 'controlled loss of control'), it is enacted in particular sociomaterial arrangements (see, for example, Dennis and Farrugia, 2017). Such trends disrupt 'the context' by twisting the focus: from human rationality within the context to one of *relationality*; from the drug effect to one of *affect*; and from the once neglected 'facilitative' drug-using *equipment* and *space and time* to constitutive elements.

Relationality

In 2013, the *International Journal of Drug Policy* launched a special issue, edited by Cameron Duff, on the use of science and technology studies, particularly, post-human and actor-network theories (mainly, as developed by John Law [2009] and Annemarie Mol [2010]), for an 'empirical revitalisation of social science in the service of explaining AOD use' (2013: 167). This edition marked a vital shift for critical drug studies in how it treats context as more-than-human and relational: a trajectory that can be plotted through

Duff's own work. In his early research, Duff conceptualises 'pleasure *in* context' (my emphasis), and a human-centred 'assemblage of risks, conscious and unconscious choices and decisions, physical and psychical sensations, affects, corporeal processes, structural and contextual forces' (2008: 385). More recently, however, Duff's sophisticated analytical skills turn to how 'social contexts may themselves be understood as discrete assemblages of such objects, spaces and actants' (Duff, 2012: 145). Drawing from actor-network theory (ANT), which refutes a subject/object binary, Duff (2009; 2011; 2012; 2013; 2014b) develops an assemblic approach to context. Following the way ANT has questioned what social scientists mean by 'the social', namely in seeing phenomenon as 'socially constructed', Duff seeks to understand AOD use 'after' context: 'bundling all of the non-human agencies together in the artifice of context merely obscures rather than explains the character of these forces, actants and processes' (2011: 404–5).

Duff (2014b) conceives of the context of AOD use as an assemblage of spaces, bodies and affects. Analysing an interview excerpt in a study on the social context of methamphetamine use in Melbourne, Australia, Duff considers what a theory of structural context might miss in an interviewee's account of methamphetamine use in the workplace. Focussing on the 'co-functioning' of space, affects and bodies, including the mundane technologies, such as the computer system, he is able to consider how these elements transformed the interviewee's activity and productivity, integral to the drug experience, which might have been overlooked in an account of political economy. Like this approach disrupts structures 'out there', Duff uses this relational, assemblic lens to disrupt an idea of rationality 'in here'. 'Singling out one actor in this network – such as the consuming subject – without acknowledging the agency of the myriad additional actors involved in this consumption merely reinforces the quaint dogma of rational choice' (Duff, 2012: 155). In de-centring the human, contexts come to constitute these more-than-human experiences, including non-human materiality and forces as well as the skin, neurotransmitters, nervous system, feelings and emotions.

Affect

Following turns to relationality, social scientists have come to understand drug contexts in terms of affects rather than effects. In a recent essay by Frederik Bøhling (2017), he accounts for pleasure as affect. Affects are generated by assemblages or 'socio-material arrangements that are simultaneously ordering and changing the social field in patterned processes of becoming-other (Deleuze and Guattari, [1987]), or more simply put, our dynamic cultural and physical contexts' (Bøhling, 2017: 136). Drug events, here hallucinogenic 'trips', are seen to move and be moved by affects not solely of the substance, consumer or context, but a complex intra-action of all three. By conceptualising the drug effect, pleasure, as an affect, it too produces new subjectivities and becomings rather than being an end point, a closing down of affect. These ideas mature from an earlier study in which Bøhling uses Duff's (2012; 2014a) notion of the 'assemblage' – as bodies, forces, affects – to account for the pleasures enacted in the nightclub so that the drug-using subject is always 'intricately entangled in their environs of other people, norms, music, lights, and smell' (2014: 387). He notes

> academic and political conceptions of AOD use and nightlife which attend solely to the rational and deliberate faculties of the human subject miss a large part of social (night)life that is driven by or embedded in forces below, beyond or intertwined with the cognitive mind.
>
> (Bøhling 2014: 385–6)

Bøhling identifies the atmospheric of the crowd to be particularly important: 'a crowded context for some of my participants was a vital part of the club assemblage, co-constituting (and enhancing) the musical, social and chemical pleasures on offer in the club' (2014: 377). Affect, therefore, moves an account of drugs both away from effects as end points, as well as cognitive rationality and control.

In another related way, Duff and Moore (2015) consider the 'affective atmosphere' of night-time 'spaces of mobility' that get people to the club, including 'fun' journeys on the tram, walking or cycling. They look at how certain atmospheres 'prime' individuals. In this sense, 'action' or 'choosing to act' is not limited to human rationality, but shared and negotiated in relation to the environment – 'how these atmospherics are modulated, compounded or resisted in encounters between bodies in transit' (2015: 311). In one of the first studies to introduce ANT to the drugs field, Demant (2009) argues that 'the enjoyment is, in other words, a matter of how the body gets enacted by the very networks in which the substance is used' (2009: 28), and, in this, attempts to 'follow how alcohol is used for enacting a pleasure-filled body' (2009: 35). In his work with colleagues on the affective space of the club (Demant et al., 2010; Demant, 2013), they challenge approaches that separate risk and pleasure:

> Anxiety, pride, anger, shame and embarrassment are embodied simultaneously with the affects of love, joy, sympathy and so on. Alcohol, illicit drugs, bouncers, music and other human or non-human actants are part of the place. It is within this heterogeneous assemblage that affects become embodied.
>
> (Demant, 2013: 196)

Through this, the authors argue that harm reduction policies should be directed towards improving affective spaces rather than a singular focus on the ingestion of substances: 'If the space of the club is approached as being more than a mono-affectual space of either risk or pleasure, then it would be possible to reduce conflicts and produce more inclusive space' (Demant, 2013: 200).

What this work on affect shows is that rather than contexts situating human actors, or even materially constituting drug effects, they are part of the very bodies that make people act and feel. More will be said on this in the next chapter, but, for now, one of the other major implications of this recent disruption to context is a more serious treatment of the material items that are usually seen as merely facilitative.

'Equipment'

Nicole Vitellone has perhaps taken 'the material' more seriously than most in this so-called 'material turn'. Through sustained attention over the last fifteen years on the technology of the syringe for understanding injecting drug use and its cultural diffractions, Vitellone's work highlights how this object creates new ways of being. In what she calls a 'syringe sociology', addicted subjectivity is not socially constructed but requires, drawing from Gomart and Hennion's (1999) seminal work on drugged attachments, the syringe (Vitellone, 2015). By turning attention away from the pre-defined social position of the user-subject, for example, as abject, which is perhaps Vitellone's biggest grievance, she says something else 'may arrive' (2015: 388). The object becomes her informant. Dissatisfied with the Bourdieu-influenced studies of injecting drug use, centred on the political economy of injecting, of which there have been many (e.g. Bourgois, 1995; 1998; Bourgois and Schonberg, 2009; Parkin, 2013; Rhodes et al., 2005; 2012), Vitellone positions the syringe as more than a conduit for social structures, but as something that is engaged by and engaging of subjects and social worlds. Instead of being embedded within hierarchies of class, gender and ethnicity, the syringe comes to mean and do different things as an agent in changing dispositifs or assemblages. For example, Vitellone carefully describes how practices of marking or scratching syringes 'are not human practices of knowing but material practices of intra-acting that enact responsibility, ethics and care', actively producing an intimate relationship with another (2017: 110–13).

Space-time

As well as disrupting the subject and object within contexts, this new material turn disrupts the idea of these contexts or spaces existing externally to time and vice versa. Time and space are shown to co-constitute. In an important article, Suzanne Fraser uses Mikhail Bhaktin's chronotype (time-space) with Karen Barad's notion of intra-action to account for how in 'the context of the methadone dosing point, time and space co-produce each other as a chronotype of the queue' (2006: 192). Ironically, the tempo-spatiality of

the queue, such as having to wait for a substantial amount of time in constrained, often stigmatised spaces (connected to methadone and vis-à-vis
opiate use) with other clients (they may wish to avoid), reproduces some
of the same tempo-spatialities as those involved in regular heroin use, e.g.
having to wait on street corners with other stigmatised opiate users. In other
words, these arrangements render methadone users in a similar space and
time as 'before'. Rather than clients entering treatment, 'the client and queue
("location, layout, staff and clients") co-construct each other', cultivating
certain behaviours and subjectivities which may not exist otherwise, such
as, Fraser notes, an incident of violence, or buying and selling methadone
to other clients.

In a very different context, of MDMA use, Farrugia (2015) explores how
spatial and temporal arrangements, such as bathtubs, 'increased the like-
lihood that the affects that emerged during MDMA consumption would
be conducive for [intimacy and] intimate communication' (2015: 248). He
explores how young men 'play' with 'space and time in bringing about new
and positive sensations, experiences, and affects', disrupting societal ex-
pectations of masculinity (2015: 240). More will be said on space-time as
we move through the book, but I flag it here to show how abstract measures of space and time have been disrupted in new understandings of
context-as-assemblage.

In this section on 'disrupting the context', I have shown how recent turns to
the material and more-than-human have disrupted anthropocentric notions
of context. Researchers have started to follow the specificity of drug events
and how they emerge through human and non-human processes. This has
shifted attention away from emplaced (in time, space) decision-making and
meaning to our relational make-up in drug-using events, to affects rather
than effects, non-human materiality as they constitute bodies rather than
merely aid them, and space and time as always made and embodied through
each other.

Bringing these three sections together, what we learn from studying drugs
in recent times is that we are always living beyond ourselves, not only living
alongside, but partially constituted through others, of which our long-term
and ubiquitous commitment to drugs (licit and illicit) surely highlights
(Dumit, 2012). 'Drug effects' cannot be traced to the choices of the user, the
essence of the substance or even 'the context' of use, but must be seen as a
complex 'intra-action' of sociomaterial matter – bodies, technologies and
forces. Therefore, it is by tracing these mattering practices in action that
new ways of knowing and doing drugs can emerge. Building on these existing post-human and new material trajectories in critical drug and addiction
studies, this book pays attention to injecting drug use and what its emergent
subjects and objects can tell us about the phenomenon and how to do it better. More than imprints of our social making (as problematisations), this is
about how injecting subjects and objects, or rather bodies (as problems) make

'trouble' (Haraway, 2016). In what ways do they 'kick back' or perhaps, even better, kick out or kick off? How can they be known in their own terms? This requires methodological and theoretical sensitivity attuned to not only the non-human, but the more-than-human. Exploring these more-than-human drug worlds or the ways drugs, bodies and worlds are mediated and mediate each other, I hope to initiate a different kind of drug study that can get to know these processes in more equal and precise terms, and thereby learn new ways of interfering and caring for them. To return again to the epigraph, drugs cannot be understood 'in extension'. Far from generalities of pleasure and misfortune, we need a closer mode of knowing. It is to this end that I propose an approach to drug use based on bodies, and more specifically, injecting drug use based on injecting bodies. Bodies are an ontologically flatter, livelier and more intricate way of engaging with the different forces at play in drug use without reducing entities and experiences to subject/object binaries that proliferate and constrain current ways of understanding and intervening. Next, I turn briefly to how these bodies made themselves known in this research project and where they appear in the book.

Chapter outline: dispersing bodies

As this introduction has shown, new (material, post-human) thinking in AOD studies has thoroughly unsettled the three cornerstones of its discipline, the 'drug, set, and setting', as Zinberg (1984) famously conceived. In a tentative attempt to put the pieces back together again, this book proposes an approach based on bodies. As humans, substances and contexts are seen to have little that inherently distinguishes them from each other, bodies, broadly conceived, as more-than-human entities, defined by their capacity to affect and be affected, become a more exacting way to understand drug-using practices and effects as they occur in the drug consumption or treatment event.

Chapter 1 explores in more detail how bodies are always in a process of becoming, or more accurately, in their relational make-up, becoming-with. The chapter details an approach to *injecting* bodies, which is as much methodological and ontological as it is theoretical and epistemological. In other words, our abilities to *know* are entangled with what can *be*. Following process and new materialist thought, bodies are brought about through their flows of desire or affect, in which how they materialise or matter is constantly changing and thus they must be studied in practice and defined by their capacity to act. It is through closer attention to bodies as affect-matter-practice that new ways of being can be revealed.

The research presented in this book is based on several months observations at a central London drug service, alongside 'creative', in-depth interviews with people who inject drugs (predominantly heroin and crack cocaine) and those who work with them including drug service workers, managers, a drug service commissioner and a doctor. Rather than trying to depict bodies, a Deleuzo-Guattarian cartography is employed as an ontologically flatter way to register those bodies that may escape our usual epistemologies. Through a method called body mapping, participants were invited to map their bodies in relation to how they were made (in relation to human and non-human others) to act, feel and think in the injecting event. Interspersed throughout the book, these hand-drawn illustrations bring to life and make possible some of the analysis as a stark reminder of the dispersed nature of injecting bodies, as they are made, or rather unmade and remade, in the injecting event. Furthermore, as these bodies are partially made in research, we become invested in what bodies to make.

Displacing thinking as the preserve of the mind, Chapter 2 explores what happens when participants think about their drug use in terms of pleasure. A paradox emerges in which pleasure is seen to be addictive, but addiction cannot be pleasurable. Unravelling the ways that 'addiction' and 'pleasure' are brought into tension in these thinking practices that are also very much material practices, pleasurable feelings are always *in touch* with not-so-pleasurable concepts. It is in this collision, or what Deleuze and Guattari call a 'zone of exchange', that it becomes impossible for participants to conceive of one without the other. However, thinking *with* pleasure (see also Race, 2017), the chapter argues that wider discussions of how drugs are experienced (which can include pleasure amongst many other affects or ways of feeling, thinking and acting) can take place in drug-treatment practice and policy.

Chapter 3 explores how drug affects, such as pleasure, following on from the previous chapter, come to be felt in the injecting event itself. In rethinking Howard Becker's (1953) classical learning theory in light of Latour's (1999a) and Gomart and Hennion's (1999) 'sociology of attachment', the chapter considers pleasure as a relational achievement (see also Race, 2008; Vitellone, 2015). Far from an individual or subjective matter, it is one shared amongst a range of bodies, technologies and forces, including substances, paraphernalia, peers, space and time. Participants provide detailed accounts of how they work within sociomaterial collectives to open themselves up to a necessary passivity for the injecting assemblage to work, to be taken in a pleasurable way. But due to the precarious nature of the injecting event, the assemblage can easily shift. Or, to use one participant's metaphor of the 'tilting glass of water', the glass can slip, and one's precious load lost. Participants engage in these attuned and attuning practices within these collectives, but are still never fully in control. In this sense, unlike previous accounts of injecting pleasure as a 'rush' (Vitellone, 2003b), pleasure gets expressed as 'success', accounting for both a rush and relief at the injecting assemblage coming together. This is a fragile affair contingent on a collaborative balancing act of bodies, technologies and forces. The 'speedball' injection, a simultaneous injection of heroin and crack cocaine, in many ways epitomises this balancing act. Revered by my interlocutors as the 'ultimate high', if done correctly, the 'speedball' – its infrastructure and affects – could bring about an intense pleasure of feeling both 'up' and 'down'.

Chapter 4 investigates where bodies were becoming-with drugs in a different way. For some participants, drug use had become a vital part of their lives, that is, for living: for becoming 'normal', 'healthy' or 'better' and 'other' versions of themselves. Drawing from Deleuze, amongst other vitalist philosophers, the chapter conceives of life as a force, and how 'forms' are brought into being through these processes. As bodies are something we *do*, it looks at how drugs for some participants had become part of their very embodiment – for 'keeping oneself together' – which made giving them up an undesired, even impossible task. Furthermore, taking a Deleuzian notion of health (Duff, 2014a) as the 'power of acting', drugs, for some, were intimately entangled with becoming healthier as participants described benefits to both mental and physical health. This disrupts normative thinking on drug use as harmful. Rather than drugs being about destroying life, they were part of sustaining, even enhancing life. But in these events, drug-using bodies can also connect to bodies with 'stratifying tendencies', such as the 'junkie image' (Malins, 2004), which blocks some ways of becoming-other, explored here through devastating accounts of stigma and marginalisation. Instead of there being any simple causal relation between drugs and the 'human' body as harmful or indeed pleasurable, bad (as well as good) drug effects are very much entangled within assemblages of technologies, forces and bodies, including in some cases legal bodies and oppressive bodies of knowledge.

Chapter 5 'troubles' the UK drug policy of 'recovery'. Considering the different ways injecting bodies become-together in the book – as rush-relief, life sustaining, enhancing, blocking – this chapter disrupts a reliance on simplified and abstracted governance based on illicit drugs as intrinsically bad and in need of abstention. Introducing the concept of habit, injecting bodies are seen to become habituated through a repetitive process of thinking, acting and feeling. Drawing largely from service providers' accounts of 'movement', this chapter looks at how intervention practices worked *with* these habits. These enactments of 'movement' go against a prescriptive notion of 'movement towards abstinence' seen to define the 'recovery agenda'. Where recovery is premised on detachable relations, namely separating 'the drug' from 'the body' in abstention, these practices were happening with a deeper appreciation for relations and the ways bodies become-with drugs. Mediating these drug-body-world relations, service providers attuned to these habituated collectives, moving in 'slower' and 'smaller' ways. To use Donna Haraway's concept of 'staying with the trouble', workers troubled recovery by engaging with an alternative form of intervention that refused absolute ways of knowing drug-using bodies and doing drug treatment (or re-covering bodies). Working with habits enacts a more intimate form of caring for injecting bodies on their own terms (as they make themselves known) in what workers called 'harm reduction and *more*' (to emphasise the movement). By bringing epistemology in touch with ontology, ethics in touch with politics and injecting bodies in touch with other bodies, more-than-harm reduction offers an approach to producing wider sensitivity and 'response-ability' (Barad, 2012; Haraway, 2008) in a time when injecting bodies are most literally failing to matter.

The book concludes by drawing together these different sociomaterial injecting bodies as they have dispersed through the chapters and speculates on how we might be able to bring 'better' (in terms of their capacity to affect and be affected) bodies into being. Revisiting Barad's idea of making 'matter *matter*', the chapter explores how bodies are 'cut together-apart' in practice and thus how they can be crafted in more empowering ways (to use Deleuze's notion of 'power of acting'). It looks at the way bodies are drawn, or rather undrawn and redrawn (literally, in the body maps), disrupting binary thinking that has dominated how we understand and intervene with drug use based on addiction/pleasure, activity/passivity, health/harm and harm reduction/recovery. By acknowledging our role (as researchers, practitioners, policymakers) alongside others (people who use drugs, legal bodies, knowledge systems, substances, 'paraphernalia', harm reduction technologies, etc.) in making boundaries, we can help to bring bodies together differently, more care-fully and response-ably (Barad, 2012). Unlike previous constructionist accounts of social forces disciplining a defenceless body, this approach is about allowing bodies to make themselves known through our collective ability to respond to them. This involves practices of mediation and working *with* bodies, that is, within *the tensions* in thinking bodies, *the attachments* in practising bodies, *the flows* of desire in living bodies, and *the habits* in intervening-with bodies in drug treatment, to make injecting bodies better.

Notes

1   Askew (2016) recently draws from the framework to conceptualise adult (over thirty years old) drug taking as 'functional fun'. The fact that the book has been updated (Aldridge et al., 2011) speaks to its influence and success. See Measham and Shiner (2009) for reflections on this 'legacy'.

2   Tim Rhodes and others have promoted a socially produced account of how people make decisions in light of and to mediate the risks associated with drug use (indeed the premise of the *International Journal of Drug Policy*, edited by Rhodes, is to platform these very issues).

3   For summaries of this move in geography, see Anderson and Wylie (2009), Jackson (2000), Anderson and Tolia-Kelly (2004), Rose and Wylie (2006), and Whatmore (2006). In anthropology, the material turn – in the sense that it is linked to Deleuze, Stengers, Strathern and ANT – has been more commonly

known as the 'ontological turn'; see Somatosphere (2014–2015) for a series of guides. In sociology, see Preda (1999) and Pierides and Woodman (2012). In science and technology studies, see Woolgar et al. (no date).

4 Professor Nutt was famously dismissed from the Advisory Council for the Misuse of Drugs for comparing the harms of ecstasy use to horse riding.

5 The National Institute on Drug Abuse, based in the US, is a key proponent of the brain disease model of addiction, and funds the vast majority of the world's research on drug use and addiction.

Chapter I

Approaching bodies
'Becoming-with'

> We believe in a world in which individuations are impersonal, and singularities are pre-individual.
>
> Gilles Deleuze, 1994: xix

The ideas presented in this book are made possible and held together by a relational ontology. Inspired by the work of Gilles Deleuze (and Félix Guattari), amongst others, this is the idea that bodies are not separate from the world but immanent to it, constituted with the world, and thus in a constant state of flux. *Bodies are always in a process of becoming.* With this, I hope to bring bodies to the forefront of a sociological study of drugs, to inject them, so to speak, where they have been historically neglected. As Thomas and Ahmed argue, 'the body has traditionally been a marginal presence in sociology, owing to the Cartesian binaries that became entrenched in the early developments of the discipline' (2004: 3). Furthermore, sociology has positioned itself against biological models (like addiction or a reductive understanding of the body's chemical response to drugs), and consequently, a focus on the material body has been treated with suspicion (Shilling, 2012: 45–76). Therefore, as seen in the Introduction, sociological research on alcohol and other drugs (AOD) has tended to favour a 'rationalising' and 'social' approach to making sense of people's seemingly irrational or dependent behaviour to consume drugs that have been marked as harmful. As 'recreational' AOD use – drug taking which is seen to be without dependency, often at the weekend, and for social cohesion – is easier to fit into these frames, this is what has dominated our sociological imagination. This project, on the other hand, seeks to redress this neglect of those drugs and drug practices deemed dependent, addictive or problematic and thus as less interesting to the sociological gaze in order to complicate drug effects to the point that such categorisations make little sense and a more entangled and intimate understanding is reached. But, in saying this, I do not mean to reinvigorate a commitment to the physical body ('body we have') or phenomenological body ('body we feel') as individually bounded, which is perhaps partially responsible for this broader disinterest in the body. Rather, I hope to invoke a flatter understanding of bodies (in the plural), or, as Latour (2004a) aptly phrases, the 'interesting body', which is always in relation to others, and defined through this relationality, in its capacity to affect and be affected.

The Deleuzian concept of 'becoming' disrupts a Platonic 'being', so that the world does not start with forms but connections, and thus, *bodies* rather than subjects and objects. 'In shifting from a model of Being to becoming there is a move away from placing the subject-object binary at the core of an analysis of the world, and a conception instead of the centrality of bodies' (Guillaume and Hughes, 2011: 150). Deleuze's philosophy is based on life or desire as a machinic force. This life source is produced by and producing of bodies, so that a force for life and bodies occur simultaneously. 'Desire is always assembled and fabricated, on a plane of immanence or of composition which must itself be constructed at the same time as desire assembles and fabricates' (Deleuze and Parnet, 2007: 103). Bodies are *immanent* with the world and not prior to it. Therefore, Deleuze (and with Guattari) uses the concept of the 'body without organs' to help imagine a body beyond its assumed boundaries – a body not made up of blood, organs, bones, etc., but 'always extending beyond itself and being conjoined with or articulated by practices, technologies, institutions, objects and so on' (Blackman, 2008: 110). Bodies in this sense are considered 'desiring machines', that is, they are always in connection with others, gaining their ability to affect and be affected from this relationality.

In the famous example from *A Thousand Plateaus*, Deleuze and Guattari describe how a wasp and orchid, in pollination, are immanent to each other. There is 'a becoming-wasp of the orchid and a becoming-orchid of the wasp' (1987: 10). Their capacities to act (affect and be affected) come about through each other, as the wasp becomes part of the orchid's reproductive system and the orchid becomes part of the wasp's nutritional intake, any perceived boundaries are broken down and new ones emerge. As an assemblage, there is what Deleuze and Guattari call a deterritorialisation and reterritorialisation – 'the two becomings interlink and form relays in a circulation of intensities' (Deleuze and Guattari, 1987: 10). In these (re)assemblings, something different emerges, a wasp-orchid or orchid-wasp. This is seen as a 'becoming-with' or 'becoming-together'. Following Haraway, '[i] f we appreciate the foolishness of human exceptionalism then we know that becoming is always becoming *with*, in a contact zone where the outcome, where who is in the world, is at stake' (Haraway, 2008: 244, original emphasis).

For the purposes of this book, this includes 'becoming-with drugs' (Michael and Rosengarten, 2012). In Mike Michael and Marsha Rosengarten's (2012) introduction to a special issue of *Body & Society,* looking at 'medicine's bodies', 'becoming' is considered in relation to 'eventuation'. That is, each event produces new becomings. In summarising Cooper's

(2012) work on bodies in the pharmaceutical marketplace, Michael and Rosengarten use the concept of 'becoming-with drugs' to include pharmaceutical companies in how people come to experiment with (pharmaceutical) drugs – how they become-together. Here, I employ the term to explore the injecting event and assemblages, which contain illicit as well as licit drugs alongside those institutions, technologies, knowledges, etc., that make certain ways of being-with drugs possible.

'Becoming-with' is significant as it highlights the joint make-up of entities, not as separate interacting components but always together, in their making, that is, a difference-in-itself, or in Haraway's (2003; 2008) terms a relationality 'all the way down'. Therefore, my starting point is always with 'intra-acting' bodies rather than interacting bodies. Coined by Karen Barad (2003; 2007), the term highlights a relationality within bodies rather than between them. Where an 'interaction' suggests an encounter between two predefined bodies, an 'intra-action' acknowledges the relationality of those bodies that are pre-individually relational, or what Blackman and Venn call a 'conjoining of thoroughly entangled processes' (2010: 9). Furthermore, according to Barad, separations between bodies, or 'cuts', are produced through their sociomaterial intra-action. Living singularly is always a product of multiplicity. This begs the questions: How do we *do* injecting bodies? And how can we *do* them better (e.g. in drug research, treatment and policy)?

Affect, matter, practice

Before turning to these two key structuring questions of the book, which will be addressed in the chapters to come, I wish to explain how they came about. This relies on three inter-related conceptual moves. First, as seen, affect is central to the immanence that brings bodies into being, which rethinks agency, experience and embodiment. Second, if matter is always in immanence (becoming), matter is by no means given, but is *made to matter* (which ties epistemology to ontology, and politics to empiricism). Third, if bodies are made to matter, we must look at the practices by which they come about. And, if matter is made to matter through onto-epistemological practices, we are all implicated. The book, therefore, attempts to trace this mattering and where injecting bodies could be made to matter more.

Affect

> We know nothing about a body until we know what it can do, in other words, what its affects are, how they can or cannot enter into composition with other affects, with the affects of another body, either to destroy that body or to be destroyed by it, either to exchange actions and passions with it or to join with it in composing a more powerful body.
>
> Gilles Deleuze and Félix Guattari, 1987: 257

Over the last decade there has been a movement within the humanities and social sciences towards 'affect' (Clough and Halley, 2007). This can be seen as a response to dominant paradigms of representation and discourse that have failed to take bodily experiences seriously beyond these sites. This is particularly pertinent to a project on drugs and their effects, which are clearly of the body, but yet rarely examined in sociology as such (noteworthy exceptions were included in the Introduction). According to Deleuze (and Guattari) and Latour, through Spinoza, bodies are defined by their ability to affect and be affected, which thoroughly disrupts an idea of bodily essence and 'the body' as autonomous.

> L'affect (Spinoza's affectus) is an ability to affect and be affected. It is a prepersonal intensity corresponding to the passage from one experiential state of the body to another and implying an augmentation or diminution in that body's capacity to act.
>
> (Deleuze and Guattari, 1987: xvi)

A theory of affect displaces the rational individual and the Cartesian body/ mind dichotomy, and for these reasons, is crucial to this project for rethinking three important fields in particular: *agency, experience* and *embodiment*.

Affects transcend the individual and environment. In Deleuzian terms, the virtual is infolded in the actual: 'actualization belongs to the world of the virtual' (Deleuze and Parnet, 2007:149). This broadens human agency beyond an individual navigating through their environment. In this, it similarly displaces the biological and the social. 'Affects aren't feelings [or emotions], they're becomings that spill over beyond whoever lives through them (thereby becoming someone else)' (Deleuze, 1995b: 137). For Latimer and Meile, affects draw attention to 'how people and things are moved about, and even transformed' (2013: 8). Affects work in-between, beyond and through bodies. 'That's what it's like on the plane of immanence: multiplicities fill it, singularities connect with one another, processes or becomings unfold, intensities rise and fall' (Deleuze, 1995b: 146–7).

Affects are what 'move' bodies (in their becoming), and in this, determine how they are able to be moved and move others. Affects are essential to agency, how bodies simultaneously affect and are affected, and thus agency, is inherently linked to relationality rather than autonomy. In reference to Spinoza, Massumi writes:

> He talks of the body in terms of its capacity for affecting or being affected. These are not two different capacities – they always go together. When you affect something, you are at the same time opening yourself up to being affected in turn, and in a slightly different way than you might have been the moment before.
>
> (2015: 3–4)

But this grasp of agency through affect modulation is not just about what bodies can do, but also how they are curtailed by what they cannot do. Such dynamism comes about through patterns of territorialisation and deterritorialisation, which thoroughly disrupts a distinction between the individual and structure (Deleuze and Parnet, 2007; Deleuze and Guattari, 1987). Where deterritorialisation produces movement, reterritorialisation brings assemblages back into order or organisation. There is a permanent movement between 'coding and mutation' (Deleuze and Parnet, 2007: 146). Assemblages are made up of three kinds of lines: molar lines that 'form a segmentary, circular, binary, aborescent system'; molecular lines, in which 'the line no longer forms a contour, and instead passes *between* things, *between* points... the multiplicity it constitutes is no longer subordinated to the One'; and lines of flight that carry the assemblage or territory away (Deleuze and Guattari, 1987: 505, original emphasis). Where molar lines organise, and molecular lines free up assemblages, a 'line of flight' can start something new – 'deterritorialisation is the movement by which "one" leaves the territory' (Deleuze and Guattari, 1987: 508).

Affects recalibrate experience and cognition beyond the individual self. Deleuze's philosophy of 'transcendental empiricism' starts with experience, but an experience that is not confined to the individual. That is, human subjectivity or consciousness is seen as always part of the outside (Deleuze, 1994). Empiricism is transcendental: it is not about 'being', it is not about matter, reality, man, consciousness or even 'the world' (Colebrook, 2002: xxix). Again, it is about immanence – 'transcendence is always a product of immanence' (Deleuze, 1995a: 388), or even, what could be called intra-action. *One* is always a product of multiplicity. Experience is 'the passage from one sensation to another [...] but as becoming, as an increase or decrease in power (virtual quantity)' (Deleuze, 1995a: 384). This is not limited to human experience, but includes the experiences of all sorts of machines, including animals and plants (Colebrook, 2002: xxix). In this sense, we need to take seriously the vitality of non-human things (see e.g. Bennett, 2010). For Clough (2009), this expanded empiricism, or what she calls 'infra-empiricism', 'allows a rethinking of bodies, matter and life through new encounters with visceral perception and pre-conscious affect' (2009: 44). This goes beyond what we see and hear, to other ways of experiencing, such as tuning in or 'attuning' to becomings, where the virtual and actual meet. 'Attunement' offers a different way of knowing (onto-epistemologically) as part of these sociomaterial collectives we study.

To sum up so far, affect is central to a relational account of injecting bodies for it takes agency and experience seriously whilst seeing them as thoroughly entangled (sociomaterial) processes. Following this sentiment, it also disrupts normative ideas of embodiment. To be embodied is not in any way to be separated from the 'outside'. Indeed, embodiment is the very task of living singularly in the face of multiplicity (Blackman, 2012). The body is always pre-individually relational, or what Blackman (2012) refers to as a matter of brain-body-world entanglement, or even, for this study, drug-body-world entanglement (Dennis, 2016). Where some accounts of embodiment suggest a separation of both the individual and environment, or mind and body, in, for example, 'reflecting on' the body, seeing bodies as intra-acting suggests something else. Summarised in Pink's sensorial methodology:

> The distinction between sensation and intellect that is implied by the idea that one might define a corporeal experience by reflecting on it and giving it meaning proffers a separation between body and mind and between doing (or practice) and knowing.
>
> (2009: 23)

When we separate the corporeal in this way, we are presupposing a distinction that is not there. The same can be said when the corporeal is neglected in favour of the rationalising mind. For example, in valuing the social reasons *behind* drug use and the consequential meaningfulness of their effects, such as pleasure, the embodied affects become largely overlooked as a product of the physical body. For Pink, 'this implies the objectification of the corporeal experience by the rational(ising) mind' (2009: 24). Instead, what a theory of affect allows is an account of bodies beyond these boundaries, defined more broadly by their capacity to affect and be affected or a 'power of acting' (Deleuze, 1992). Cameron Duff (2014a) expands on this definition in his account of health and illness. Health, he says, 'may be understood to involve those forms of bodily activity that extend a body's range of action' (2014a: 75).

Taking Duff's concept of health forward here, as a Deleuzian 'power of acting' (2014a: 135), some bodies are brought together in productive ways, where in other assemblages there are delimitations, which can be brought about through both territorialisation and deterritorialisation. By mapping these bodies through the pages of this book, I consider where these powers expand and contract. Research and intervention then becomes about interfering within these connections, to increase capacities to act, and above all, to avoid creating new blockages, which, as Deleuze stresses, is only too easy: 'It is precisely the whole group of body organizations that will smash the plane or field of immanence, and will impose upon desire another type of plane, each time stratifying the body-without-organs' (2006: 130).

Matter

> Language matters. Discourse matters. Culture matters. There is an important sense in which the only thing that does not seem to matter anymore is matter.
>
> Karen Barad, 2003: 801

In this well-cited extract, Karen Barad highlights how, for a long time, especially during the 1990s, body studies had become preoccupied with discourse and culture. Informed chiefly by a Foucaultian turn, researchers sought to understand bodies as 'docile', inscribed by discourse and cultural semiotics. As such, these bodies were often *done to* rather than *doing*. In other words, they were often made immaterial, or inconsequential to the discourses that controlled or contained them. In reinstating the body as matter that *matters*, Barad sought to shake up this over-reliance on discourse.[1] In her eminent essay, *Posthumanist Performativity: Toward an Understanding of How Matter Comes to Matter*, Barad positions discourse and matter as co-constituting, and argues: 'What is needed is a robust account of the materialization of *all* bodies – 'human' and 'nonhuman' – and the material-discursive practices by which their differential constitutions are marked' (2003: 810, original emphasis).

Developed further in *Meeting the Universe Halfway*, her philosophy of 'agential realism' speaks to this pursuit.

> I propose 'agential realism' as an epistemological-ontological-ethical framework that provides an understanding of the role of human and nonhuman, material and discursive, and natural and cultural factors in scientific and other social-material practices, thereby moving such considerations beyond the well-worn debates that pit constructivism against realism, agency against structure, and idealism against materialism.
>
> (2007: 26)

Intra-actions of discourse and matter are 'cut together-apart' (Barad, 2012). These 'cuts' are social-material or rather as I prefer sociomaterial.[2] Their very separation is a matter of their togetherness. That is, 'all bodies, not merely "human" bodies, come to matter through the world's iterative intra-activity' (Barad, 2003: 823). 'Intra-action' does a number of things for this project and for understanding the extent of bodies' entanglements with drugs, technology and world-making more generally. First, it cements matter as social *and* material. Second, it highlights that the apparatuses through which bodies are known or come to 'matter' are intimately linked to their ontological existence, which requires new modes of 'knowing' within these entanglements. Third, it reaffirms what we know from 'affect', that what bodies can *do* is a matter of relationality, and therefore, we need to map these bodies in practice.

Barad (2007) rethinks performativity through the work of quantum physicist Niels Bohr. In revolutionising a Newtonian physics, Bohr shows that whether an electron is a particle or wave is dependent on the testing apparatus. Extending this to social theory, reality and the practices and frames for which it is known are entangled in what Barad calls an onto-epistemology. The term 'enactment' is consequently used to stress the material aspect, beyond the social, in how reality comes to matter through intra-active 'cuts'. Rather than a Cartesian cut, intra-active cuts do not assume a prior separation between subjects and objects, mind and matter (2003: 815). Following Bohr, 'phenomena' is used to account for this entanglement of words and things, matter and meaning, objects and subjects: 'the inseparability of "observed object" and "agencies of observation"' (Barad, 2003: 814). This agential realism disrupts causality – rather than cause/effect being a matter of subjects and objects, to be objectively known, they are already entangled. Drug affects and embodiments are, therefore, phenomena that come into being through intra-acting agencies. *Matter comes to matter* through the iterative intraactivity of the world in its becoming' (2003, 823, original emphasis).

Bodies are brought into being and delimited in their being through their relationality with others. They are cut together-apart. It is therefore necessary to look at this relationality in order to make sense of the singularities and e/affects – such as drugs, bodies, pleasure, harm, etc. To add to the previous section on affect, embodiment then is also a matter of intra-action. Whilst 'embodiment' has been an overused, even abused term in sociology (when used to distance certain experiences or those experiencing it from what is deemed to be rational), it is still of value in highlighting processes of living singularly in multiplicity as only ever a partial whole. Bodies are constituted through relations or assemblages of bodies, which includes non-human bodies, for example, drugs, illicit and licit, 'paraphernalia', drug policies, technologies and so on. This approach allows for an appreciation of the *things* traditionally overlooked in sociology and the forms and objects they enact.[3] For Barad, this requires a different way of knowing or doing theory, a more embodied way. She says: 'doing theory requires being open to the world's aliveness, allowing oneself to be lured by curiosity, surprise, and wonder. Theories are not mere metaphysical pronouncements on the world from some presumed position of exteriority' (2012: 207).

In this sense, 'all life forms (including inanimate forms of liveliness) *do* theory' (Barad, 2012: 208, original emphasis). To this end, 'touch' is put forward as a collective way of knowing (Haraway, 2008). To touch and 'to be in touch' is to be attuned to these different forms (Barad, 2012). This is a kind of transcendental empiricism based on 'becoming-together apart'. Acknowledging that bodies are always in a process of becoming, intra-active cuts are made in their doing. Thinking with both Deleuze and Barad, bodies are always in becoming, defined by their capacity to affect and be affected, and are cut together-apart within sociomaterial entanglements. As such, it becomes crucial to map these bodies and their possibilities in practice, that is, how they are lived singularly, and come to matter, in the face of multiplicity.

Practice

> Despite participants' well-ordered reconstructions and rationalisations, actual [...] practice entails the confrontation and negotiation of utter confusion.
>
> Bruno Latour and Steve Woolgar, 1986: 36

According to science and technology studies, science must be studied 'in action' (Latour, 1987), in the making, or, in other words, in practice. In Latour's (2005a) actor-network theory, reality is seen to be made from a network of actants, human and non-human, and depending on how these are brought together in practice, for example, in the laboratory (with Woolgar, 1986), determines what emerges as 'fact' or 'truth'. Far from an objective (positivist) or subjective (social constructionist) matter, science involves a complex interplay of actants that disrupt what Latour calls this 'modern' divide (1993). For example, exploring Louis Pasteur's 'discovery' of the microbe, Latour (1988) diligently describes a network of the public hygiene movement, medical professional and colonial interests, alongside and entangled with the experimental equipment, scientists, published reports, etc. Studying science-in-practice is central to documenting how these realities come about, and thus where, in his later work, we might 'interfere' with these *things* (in what he calls a 'dingpolitiks') (Latour, 2005b).

If bodies, as I have argued, are energised through affect modulation, and come to matter through sociomaterial intra-action, they are only ever done and experienced in practice. Against a poststructuralism which, for some, has led to the death of the subject, I take seriously experience, subjectivity and sentience, but as always more than human and in flux. 'As actors come to participate in different "networks" [...] the "actors" start to differ from one network, discourse, logic, mode of ordering, practice to the other' (Mol, 2010: 260). Like above, this is a kind of post-human phenomenology, where bodies are multiple. In Mol's (2002) famous ethnography of atherosclerosis, she looks at how the atherosclerosis in the lab is different to the atherosclerosis in the doctor's consultation room, which is different from the atherosclerosis in the operating theatre, and so on. So, another question, for this book, becomes: What bodies are we talking about? And thus we see four kinds of injecting bodies emerge in the injecting and/or treatment-service event – those conceived, practised, lived and intervened-with.

Consequently, as aforementioned, an enduring question for body studies has been: 'How do we live singularity in the face of multiplicity?' (Blackman, 2012: 2). But this is not about a fragmented human body holding together, rather, as Mol points out, this is a collective effort, involving human and non-human bodies, or rather, for her, 'several people and lots of things' (2002: 25): 'the drawing together of a diversity of objects that go by a single name involves various modes of coordination [...] clinical notes, pressure measurement numbers, duplex graphs, and angiographic images' (Mol, 2002: 84).

How bodies exist singularly in multiplicity is a question that this book similarly strives to address in looking at the various ways people and 'human' experiences, such as pleasure, embodiment and harm, hold together (and fall away). For Mol, drugs users 'do a lot: their pleasure depends on [it]' (2010: 257). But again, this is a collective effort, and I look at how bodies come to be felt and experienced – capacitated and incapacitated ('power of acting') in their relations – as a matter of practice, which includes actants such as policies, media images and biotechnologies (e.g. methadone).

This active 'holding together' can be seen in light of a notion of habit, as proposed by Deleuze (1994) and Massumi (2002), and most recently taken up by Latour (2013). Habits expose the infolded inner and outer worlds or what others have called 'embankments' (Povinelli, 2018) in 'becoming' through practice. These are the unconscious parts of living that get built up in moving through life that are essential to it, but rarely get noticed. Seemingly inspired by Deleuze (1994), habit, for Latour, is said to be a 'mode of existence with a paradoxical hiatus that produces immanence' (2013: xii). For Latour, habit is a kind of network that allows us to live with apparent stability and continuity: 'without habit, we would never have dealings with essences, but always with discontinuities. The world would be unbearable' (Latour, 2013: 268). In this sense, it is a crucial 'mode of existence' – central to how we live singularly in the face of multiplicity – to actualise as one, in learning to be affected and affect. Latour's (2013) most recent philosophical project looks for ways to handle these multiple ontologies in a 'common world', which he says is vital for being able to deal with complexities such as the ecological crisis.

In a 'modern' world that refuses its own multiplicity, there are often conflicts. For people who use drugs, especially those who inject, this is felt intensely, as they visibly disrupt the autonomous individual – they highlight a profound 'learning to be affected' – which is pathologised and distanced from the 'modern' subject as addiction. In the coming chapters, I look at three areas of practice: the practices of habit or 'becoming-with drugs'; the scientific and drug service practices which exclude these differences in defining drug use as just one thing; and the more collective 'democratic' practices or 'interferences' that are also taking place. I end the book by suggesting ways we might be able to better engage with these practices in enabling new habits or ways of becoming-with drugs.

To recapitulate, I have approached bodies as always becoming-with. Injecting bodies are done through sociomaterial practices, but crucially this involves our own research practices and bodies. As Barad says: 'To theorize is not to leave the material world behind and enter the domain of pure ideas where the lofty space of the mind makes objective reflection possible.

Theorizing, like experimenting, is a material practice' (Barad, 2007: 55). Therefore, to approach bodies *as* always 'becoming-with' is to also say *by* becoming-with. As such, 'approaching bodies' is an inherently methodological practice, a practice that involves registering bodies in new ways.

Becoming-with as method

Injecting bodies as a methodology is about becoming-with bodies – to register them and be registered by them in new ways. To pay attention to affect, and thus the modulations of affect in constantly (sociomaterially) changing bodies, we must also become affected. We must attune to our research subjects, objects and relations. Clough refers to an 'expanded empiricism', whilst others have talked about moving from 'matters of concern' to 'matters of affect' (Latimer and Meile, 2013). Where human and non-human relations, and natural and cultural worlds, can no longer be separated in the way they once were, we must allow ourselves to be moved by these 'naturecultural' (Haraway, 2003; Latimer and Meile, 2013), more-than-human formations (Whatmore, 2013). There is no 'nature' untouched by 'culture' and vice versa (Haraway, 1991). In getting to know these new 'worlds in common', as Latour (2004b) says, we require new methods. This is 'a world that methods concerned with human interpretation and meaning cannot reach' (Adkins and Lury, 2009: 8). Unlike a 'simple empiricism', an expanded empiricism, following Deleuze, is about being able to register those life processes that go beyond consciousness: 'In fact, consciousness expresses itself only by being reflected on a subject which refers it to its objects. This is why the transcendental field cannot be defined by the consciousness which is nonetheless coextensive with it, but which eludes revelation' (Clough, 2009: 62). As such, new kinds of relating are needed to register these forms of becoming-with non-human things and more-than-human processes otherwise neglected in traditional sociological accounts of drug use.

It struck me, when I first started looking for alternative ways to study drug-using bodies and experiences such as pleasure beyond that which can be rationalised, just how few attempts there had been. Like much of our social scientific phenomena, drug use continues to be studied predominantly through that which can be verbalised in the in-depth interview despite many researchers complaining of the difficulties people have in talking about drug-using experiences. Demant states: 'when studying bodily experience like taking drugs… it is hard for the actors to verbalise what is going on' (2009: 31). Even though authors have specifically implored others to study drugged bodies and affects beyond the representational and human (as seen in the Introduction), there is often not a proposed methodological way of doing so other than through what can be consciously, cognately and verbally described. This lack of methodological imagination has been noted by Thrift (2000) in relation to the 'cultural turn' more generally in which he argues social researchers have 'allied themselves with a number of qualitative methods [and…] the narrow range of sensate life they register' (2000: 60). Wanting to extend this life, I approach method as a lively encounter, and attempt to 'notice' (Stewart, 2007) the previously unsaid and unsayable – allowing myself to be moved by the intensities, forces, sensations and affects – and the small details and materialities that often get neglected in narrative accounts.

In *Ordinary Affects*, Kathleen Stewart (2007) uses the method of 'noticing' as a way of getting closer to the 'live surface' of the ordinary – the potentiality that animates these forms – the sensations, intensities and textures, through which ordinary life is experienced (Coleman and Ringrose, 2013: 4). I use the term here in relation to noticing bodies, that is, bodies that exceed representation, and an alertness to the material sensations and affects they produce and receive, but also the invisible and immaterial forces, or the draws and pulls that compel bodies together and pull them apart. 'Bodies' is used here in its widest sense, to include human and non-human entities, and thus embodiment as a relational enactment. For me, this noticing happened alongside a Deleuzo-Guatarrian cartography. Mapping allows a flexibility towards these new formations of human and non-human processes, always in becoming, to map how they happen, or how they 'dwell' together, in forming 'worlds in common' (Latour, 2004b). But unlike past attempts at empiricism, like positivism, this empiricism not only 'captures', but also 'creates' reality (Coleman and Ringrose, 2013; Law, 2004; Law and Urry, 2004; Lury and Wakeford, 2012).

Taking bodies as assemblages that are done in practice (learning to affect and be affected), mapping is essential to grasp how they are done in relation to others and how they are made to act, feel and think through the injecting event, but notably how they could also be done differently as affects shift. Trying to identify these movements in coming together and falling away – the work required to keep them together and the fragile fault lines in breaking them apart and the traces left behind – became a fundamental part of 'noticing' where drugs were experienced positively or negatively, and where to intervene. In this section, I lay out how I went about this process – mapping *interviews*, *drawing* and *observations* together in understanding how bodies, in their constant flux, are done and could be done differently.

'Creative' interviews with people who inject drugs

The 'creative interview', coined by Jennifer Mason (2010), defines an in-depth semi-structured interview that produces additional types of data beyond the spoken word. With 'inventive methods' (Lury and Wakeford, 2012) in mind, I use the term to identify the interviewing process as both creative in its undertaking, but also creative in the realities it enacts. I attune to the interview as an affective encounter and to the affective encounters of my participants, that is, their attunements or connections with non-human things, objects, technologies and forces, for example, drugs, paraphernalia, mobile phones and certain spaces. This method allowed me to take the non-cognitive and non-rational aspects of drug use seriously where it might otherwise be dismissed as 'addiction' or 'dependency'.

If, like Hickey-Moody, we take 'affect' as a 'visceral prompt' or 'what moves us' (2013: 79), to follow affect, to become affected and affect in our research, means both to become-with participants' bodies in their registering (and production), but also to notice the ways participants are moved beyond consciousness, rationality and individuality in what is frequently 'black boxed' as addiction or dependency. Such concepts hide these nuances and intricacies of drug relations – the forces, pulls and charges between human and non-human bodies – within a singular object (Fraser, 2016; Pienaar et al., 2015). Like Stewart's rejection of 'totalized systems', this is not to say they are wrong, but 'to bring them into view as a scene of immanent force, rather than leaving them looking like dead effects imposed on an innocent world' (2007: 1). Through 'affect', new understandings can be born: 'through this conceptual lens, embodied relations mapped by research and aesthetic responsiveness can be seen as a way of constructing new imaginings of the social' (Hickey-Moody, 2013: 85).

Recruitment for the interviews initially took place through two drug services, the Dunswell and the Eastford service (pseudonyms), in two different areas of central London. I put up posters and left flyers in the waiting rooms and needle exchange areas. Recruitment also came to rely more than I anticipated on word of mouth and participants passing on flyers to their friends and acquaintances. This meant that I started attracting people to the study that lived outside the vicinity of the two services, and five participants were not using drug services at all. In total, I interviewed thirty-two people, of which thirty were currently injecting heroin and/or crack cocaine (defined as within the last four weeks). This included twenty-one men and eleven women, from a range of ethnic and social backgrounds, aged between twenty-eight and sixty years old. Of those currently injecting, fifteen participants injected heroin (with six also smoking crack cocaine), thirteen injected heroin with crack cocaine (known as 'speedball') and two injected pharmaceutical heroin or diamorphine. Although not all the participants feature in this book, they all informed it in some way (a brief participant list is provided in Appendix I).

The interviews lasted from 40 minutes to 2.5 hours, with the majority lasting approximately 1.5 hours. I conducted second interviews with four of the participants due to the interview being unfinished at the time they had to leave for another appointment. In the interview, I used a very loose topic guide, which changed iteratively to prompt discussion. I usually started by asking participants about their drug use history, then their current drug use – using a body mapping task to expand on the injecting event – how their drug use had changed over time and then their experiences of drug services, needle exchanges and opiate substitution. I was keen to explore descriptions and somatically felt experiences in order to draw out the specificities and relationality of these practices rather than focussing on their meaning and reasoning (see also Bøhling, 2014; Duff, 2014b).

Body mapping

Taking a more literal approach to cartography, I invited participants in the interview to draw a picture of their body (in the normative sense) on an A1 piece of paper and use the picture to describe how they might be feeling before, during and after injecting drugs, and what may be going on around them (these maps are included throughout the book). Beyond traditional accounts of body mapping as a way of exploring embodied experiences (Art2Be, n.d.; Brett-Maclean, 2009; Dorrell, 2007; Gastaldo et al., 2012; Tarr et al., 2014), often in relation to health conditions such as HIV/AIDS, the method here provided a 'device' (Lury and Wakeford, 2012) for registering new kinds of injecting bodies, and being-with the world. It acted both as a prompt for relating to the self and others in recollecting the injecting event, and as a prompt in the here-and-now as the participant and I (with the drawing materials) created a new body and drew-together. For many participants, feelings and thoughts came easily to paper or rather with the paper. Thinking and discussion developed in the drawing as bodies became delineated in new ways. Body mapping acted not as a 'tool', but as an active part of the interview in bringing bodies into being. I will now attend to some six things that the body maps *did* for this 'kind of attentiveness to tacit forms of coexistence' (Back, 2012: 29).

First, body mapping allowed for the 'body-we-do' to be brought into the interview through activity. By employing the body, there was an added mobility, which freed-up thinking – prompting thoughts that otherwise may not have come up through disembodied talk (Back and Puwar, 2012; Buscher et al., 2011). For example, some participants said their need for drugs was purely in their head – 'a mental thing' – but once they started drawing, and perhaps, I think, by engaging the body in movement, they were able to talk about the body, and embody their past experiences in enacting the present. In this sense, it allowed a way in 'beside' (Sedgwick, 1993) the dominant addiction model, beyond a reductionist neurological or psychological understanding.

Second, the body mapping allowed body parts to become part of the discussion. Keen to show me what they were drawing, participants rolled-up sleeves and trousers, peeled-back socks, took-off shoes, pulled down/up tops and exposed plastered skin. In these acts of intimacy, participants sought to show me their veins where they were injecting, old scars and healed injecting sites, wounds and abscesses from bacterial infections, swollen limbs, feet and hands from accidentally injecting into and disrupting the lymphatic system, and one man showed me the large holes left in his upper arms by having necrotic tissue surgically removed. Some women even stretched their underwear to one side to show me the holes made by injecting repeatedly into their femoral vein. By exposing and enacting these 'biological' parts of the assemblic body, they became entangled in the interview encounter and the bodies that became knowable.

Third, the activity changed the atmosphere and attuned me to a sense of atmosphere. By requiring movement, the interview became less clinical. The transition from talking to drawing provided the space and time to stand up and move about, checking phones, getting a drink, opening/closing windows, and we would often rearrange the tables and chairs and move closer together, so I could see what the participant was doing. With the rhythms changing, the quiet periods during the drawing also helped me register atmosphere. In Stewart's words 'atmospheric attunements are palpable and sensory yet imaginary and uncontained, material yet abstract. They have rhythms, valences, moods, sensations, tempos, and lifespans' (2011: 445). The pace of the interview slowed down, allowing mumblings, singing, whistling and sighing to emerge. The city also made itself known, entering through the windows in sounds and smells of the nearby traffic, the rumblings of the trains overhead, the sirens of emergency vehicles, and the shouts and cries of the street below. I started to notice participants' feelings and connections towards the things, objects and people they drew. One man burst into song, with the delight of his heroin memories enacted on the page, whilst another became agitated by his drawing, describing the turmoil inflicted by both wanting to and not wanting to use drugs, yet another became depressed in the event, embodying the slumped position of the figure he drew.

Fourth, the body mapping prompted a different kind of thinking and communication. Literat points out, in her study using drawing with children, that 'the physical act of creation and the bodily engagement with one's environment fosters [...] a different type of cognitive process, which transcends the domain of purely cerebral thought' (2013: 88). Body mapping encouraged a more embodied way of thinking, which fits with Deleuze's philosophy of embodied thought (Guillaume and Hughes, 2011). In this, I would argue that the previously unsaid, either the unsayable or that conceived as not important, was able to make itself known. This becomes particularly relevant for affects such as pleasure that, as we saw in the Introduction, participants are frequently encouraged to reinterpret. It provided a mode of communication where participants could *show* me rather than having to *tell* me something that was difficult to put into words. This gives weight to Literat's argument that the principal objective of participatory drawing 'is to facilitate the expression of perspectives and narratives that were previously "overlooked, rejected, or silenced"' (Singhal and Rattine-Flaherty, 2006, cited in Literat, 2013: 12). Furthermore, but perhaps more surprisingly, due to the focus on 'the body', body mapping also allowed the underexplored non-human entities of the drug assemblage to emerge. This is particularly important in disrupting a usual sociological interest in the human and social influence on people's drug use. For example, Reggie, sitting back and looking on at his body map, realised he had missed something out and exclaimed 'aha, I've missed the car' (see Figure 3.2). Rather than missing out the drug dealer, he had missed out the car. The car was a central part of the scoring process and a constant go between. There is something about the drawing or the literal flatness of the paper that allows a flatter relationship between humans and non-humans (discussed further below), which would perhaps not emerge in talk alone.

Lastly, and adding to this, body mapping allowed for the complexities or messiness in participants' experiences of injecting drugs and using services – rather than inflicting order, it allowed for everything 'all in one go': 'If research participants are asked to produce something visual (such as a drawing...), this enables them to circumvent the inherent linear mode of speech – one thing leading to another – and present a set of ideas "all in one go"' (Gauntlett, 2007: 126). This resonates with Deleuze and Guattari's (1987) concept of the rhizome (to be taken up further below): 'the rhizome enables a body's relations and potentials to be thought of as connecting-up with an almost infinite number of other bodies and potentials in multiple directions' (Malins, 2004: 98). Therefore, the body maps drew attention to and articulated a vast array of intertwining elements: non-human things, objects and technologies; body parts; people; emotions, feelings, thoughts and senses; affects, movement and other forces; along with expressions and words; and temporal and spatial structurings; even politics, policies and societal norms and values. But they also gave a sense of the texture, colour, size and depth of the complexity and the magnitude of these elements in their relationality; each competing for space on the paper, disrupting any predefined hierarchy, especially that which is perceived between humans and non-humans.

To sum up on what the body mapping *did*. It brought the interview encounter to life, both in the sense of somatic vitality – the bodies that were drawn, done and talked about – but also an embodied awareness of the injecting event – the tastes, smells, forces, charges – as the coming together of various drug assemblages – drugs, cars, mobile phones, needles, blood, veins, etc. Indeed, the two become quite inseparable. Therefore, to answer Massumi's question on methodological validity posed in the Foreword to *A Thousand Plateaus*, does it work? I hope to have shown that it does:

> The question is not: is it true? But: does it work? What new thoughts does it make possible to think? What new emotions does it make possible to feel? What new sensations and perceptions does it open up in the body?
>
> (Deleuze and Guattari, 1987: xv)

Mapping bodies opened up a space for a broader understanding and expression of bodies which come to be known as they are registered with other bodies – my body, the readers body, the body of the paper, as well as the imaginings of bodies from the injecting event. Method as a kind of becoming-with or learning to become affected (Despret, 2004; Latour, 2004a) allows new ways of becoming to emerge, which, for this study, is central to moving beyond reductionist accounts of drug harms and pleasures. Next, I turn to a more mechanistic account of how interviews with service providers added to this emergent understanding of injecting bodies and their mediation in more-than-human worlds.

Interviews with service providers

I conducted interviews with ten people working in various capacities within the provision of drug treatment. For ease, I have called these participants service providers. Service providers were recruited through the same two-drug services used for recruiting people who inject drugs (PWID) – the Dunswell service, where participant observation also took place, and the Eastford service, where no participant observation took place. The interviews lasted between one and two hours, and happened in the affiliated service, with the exception of one, which happened at the university due to the worker no longer being employed by the service at the time of the interview. I recruited participants by asking them, either in person or via email, if they were willing to participate. In order to get a sense of who I wanted to speak to and what questions to ask, I waited until the majority of the PWID interviews had been conducted before interviewing service providers. The sampling then took an iterative form, with the 'data' from each one informing who I spoke to next.

First, to get a broader sense of the treatment sector, I interviewed the manager of the Eastford service and the team leader of the Dunswell service. Picking up on what they described as a movement in the services' focus towards abstinence-based recovery and rehabilitation, I next interviewed a 'recovery social worker' and the 'community care assessor' (for residential detoxification and rehabilitation) at the Dunswell service. Noticing a difference of emphasis in the treatment setting between what was considered 'clinical' (more immediate, biomedical-based interventions) or 'recovery' (longer term) work – also divided as prescribing or psychosocial work – I interviewed a clinical 'substance misuse practitioner' from the Dunswell service and a 'recovery worker' who had very recently left the Eastford service. Then, responding to a conversation I had during participant observation at the Dunswell service with the new interim manager about opiate substitution reduction policies, I asked him for a more formal interview. Wanting to explore and compare some of these changes further, I interviewed the regional director of the drug charity that runs the Eastford service to see if these policies reflected more general changes across the sector. Next, following up on the Dunswell manager's suggestion and a growing interest in funding changes, I held an interview with a representative from the borough's drug service commission. Lastly, detecting a recurring theme on the tensions between prescription and recovery work, I interviewed the prescribing doctor at the Dunswell service.

These interviews became an essential part of the methodological assemblage or becoming-with, in particular, the elements that make up the drug treatment event, but which also subtly make themselves known in the consumption event – the governmental and local policies; treatment discourses; service procedures, practices, care-planning and monitoring; treatment spaces; opiate substitutes and prescription regulations; treatment models; funding; etc. In this, I maintained an orientation to the sociomaterial 'intra-actions' in the way words, metaphors and discourses (e.g. being 'stuck' in treatment and 'parked' on methadone in policies, procedures and everyday care practices) seemed to intra-act with other bodies (of knowledge, institutional bodies, substances, assessment forms, etc.) in creating certain ways of being, for example, 'an addict' or 'service user'.

Participant-observing

Intersecting with the interviews and drawings, I conducted participant observations at the Dunswell service, a community drug service offering support for adults over the age of eighteen who identify issues with drug use. This site was chosen for its large size, with approximately 700 current clients, and high number of heroin and crack users, which are the two substances most commonly injected. It also had many harm reduction provisions, including: a needle exchange, which supplied injecting and harm reduction equipment; a harm reduction advice service; an onsite blood-borne virus nurse; an opiate substitution prescribing service with onsite doctors; and it was trialling a scheme to provide take-home naloxone (overdose reversal) kits.

Prior to starting the participant observation, for one day a week over a ten-month (October 2012–August 2013) period, I volunteered as a 'substance misuse worker' at the service. This included shadowing workers, but I was soon encouraged to take on a small case load – perhaps illustrating the rising, but not uncontroversial role of volunteers in the sector (commented on by one service provider as an example of how the sector and workforce is becoming deskilled). I regularly key-worked three service users and saw many more when covering for other workers. I started volunteering on a Friday, but this later changed to a Wednesday. This change of day proved important as it was on a Wednesday that both the team and clinical meeting occurred and I was able to take in some of the effects of recent drug policy changes to service delivery. After a gap of approximately eight months, I carried out a further six months (April–October 2014) research at the service, again volunteering for one day a week, which forms the basis of my observational reflections here. I usually arrived just before 10 am and left around 5 pm. Not wanting to get in the way, I took on various responsibilities, many of which I had learnt as a volunteer. But, wanting to affirm my new researcher role, I negotiated to not have a caseload, but instead only see clients needing a duty worker. My time at the service included: shadowing workers; helping with administration and office tasks; filling out assessment forms with new clients; key working current clients, which included completing the necessary drug tests, attendance checks with pharmacies, writing prescription recommendations to their doctors and care planning; staffing the needle exchange; attending clinical meetings and training with the onsite doctor. These everyday practices of 'being alongside' (Latimer, 2013), or to go one-step further, becoming-with, afforded a change in how I could register bodies in the interview and vice versa; in this sense, the methods worked together in making the bodies known and knowable through this affinity and affection (learning to become affected).

Rhizomatic analysis or becoming moved

Grounded theory is aspired to by many qualitative researchers, especially in public health. However, like others, I have come to think of grounded theory as arborescent (tree-like), which goes against a Deleuzian rhizomatic style of thinking. For Deleuze, the tree is the archetype of representational thinking that 'categorises the world and establishes hierarchical relationships among classes' (MacLure, 2013: 165). In contrast: '[The rhizome is defined by] principles of connection and heterogeneity: any point of a rhizome can be connected to anything other, and must be. This is very different from the tree or root, which plots a point, fixes an order' (Deleuze and Guattari, 1987: 7).

My analysis was thereby moved rhizomatically as I was taken by some of the bodies, forces and knowledges mentioned above in new and multiple directions. This becoming-together in the research encounter often started during, if not before, the interview or observation event itself. I would consider my immediate feelings and responses in my questioning. I then took field notes afterwards to capture some of these feelings. I transcribed the forty-six interviews (thirty-six with PWID and ten with service providers) as I was keen to slow down the analysis process and re-enact the interview time-space in my mind in order to annotate the spoken words as well as the more somatic and non-verbal forms of communication that were going on. This was important so not to separate the material and immaterial aspects from the verbal. Going meticulously over the transcripts, I identified aspects – an event, scene, 'thing', sense or word – that stood out, grabbed my attention and pulled me in closer (that touched me, to use Haraway and Barad's term).

For Deleuze and Guattari, 'all tree logic is a logic of tracing' (1987: 12), and interestingly, given the urge people often had to psychoanalyse the body maps, psychoanalysis is seen as the archetype of tracing, as it views things in totalised, closed-off and hierarchical systems.

> What distinguishes the map from the tracing is that it is entirely oriented toward an experimentation in contact with the real. The map does not reproduce an unconscious closed in upon itself; it constructs the unconscious. It fosters connections between fields, the removal of blockages on bodies without organs, the maximum opening of bodies without organs onto a plane of consistency.
>
> (Deleuze and Guattari, 1987: 12)

Following this, I was keen to steer clear of an analysis that took on closed frames. Rather, I was interested in the body maps as 'live surfaces' – as a 'device' for connecting the non-hierarchical movement between things, senses, affects, etc., in producing different effects. As such, they invited reflections and diffractions, and stimulated affect and feeling in unpredictable ways (see also Blackman and Venn, 2010; Walkerdine, 2010). I tried to be receptive to these feelings and use them to better understand the participants' experiences, for example, the frustrations of needing a hit but not managing to find a vein, the embarrassment, anger and humiliation of being labelled a 'junkie', the conflicts between wanting to and not wanting to use drugs. Participants often helped me to understand feelings by offering bodily comparisons, like that seen in the title of Chapter 3, where Lucy compared a missed hit to dropping a glass of water when critically dehydrated. In this sense, some of my bodily responses were elicited in the accounts, diligently following the telling, but others were not so easily trackable and would move alongside or even against the narrative. I found one interview particularly tense and had a sense of urgency throughout, which contradicted the meaning of the words spoken and their calm and coherent delivery.

Instead of coding, unbeknown at the time, I took a more Deleuzian approach to analysis, moved by the research bodies and relations.[4] I took my transcripts, theme files, body maps and field notes together, and started mapping the interactions between diverse and disperse aspects of the data and their 'lines of flight'. I found it very hard to start with any systematic approach, and so relied on my head (in-keeping with Deleuze and Guattari's [1987] notion of the rhizomatic brain) to carry the connections before starting to map them out onto paper. I started writing down some key points, which triggered others and the mapping grew. It made sense to use a pen and paper rather than a digital interface as it offered more flexibility and movement. Similarly, for Deleuze and Guattari: 'the ideal for a book would be to lay everything out on a plane of exteriority of this kind, on a single page, the same sheet: lived events, historical determinations, concepts, individuals, groups, social formations' (1987: 9).

Like the body maps themselves, the flatness of these larger analytic maps meant that bodies, technologies, forces, etc., could exist more equally and it provided a sense of openness; to make the connections and disconnections and see things in a multidirectional, non-hierarchical and non-linear way. These 'analytical maps' allowed space for not only words of different sizes, styles and colours, but also symbols, connecting lines, arrows and the inevitable crossings out and mess to exist together, in which, to quote MacLure, 'objects, utterances, institutions, bodies, fragments *relate* in an "unholy mixture" (Lecercle, 2002) rather than orderly hierarchy' (2013: 165, my emphasis).

This approach perhaps resembles something similar to Law's (2007) 'pin-board', or MacLure's 'cabinet of curiosities', which encapsulates 'coding as a particular kind of experimental assemblage' (MacLure, 2013: 165). Furthermore, the rhizome, unlike the grounded theory image of the tree, can more easily imagine change: 'it is a methodology of looking differently at connections, and, possibly, a methodology of tracing how these connections might be made differently' (Ringrose and Coleman, 2013: 125). Therefore, 'when social scientists find and map the capture, fixing and unfixing of the body and its machinic connections they offer hope and possibility for something different in the social' (Ringrose and Coleman, 2013: 142). So, for this project, mapping not only expands our understanding of drug-body-world relations, but also allows a way of thinking about how these may be *made differently*, indeed, how they may be *made better*, to produce more good affects, and ways of becoming-other.

In negotiating these theories of affect, matter and practice outlined at the start of the chapter, I seek to elucidate where bodies are constituted in their relations with others, but how there are also excesses, both between and beyond bodies. Thinking rhizomatically, with theory, rather than through theory, I look at how these theories make possible and add to the ways bodies get done in my research – intra-acting with structures, discourse, institutions, images etc. – in becoming-with drugs. Thinking with Deleuze (and Guattari) and Barad and others from science and technology studies (STS), the book considers the coming-together of bodies, not simply by equal chance, as perhaps a purely symmetrical study might infer, but how some ways of becoming are also made more possible than others.

Ethicopolitics or doing research with care

If bodies are done differently and only held together singularly in practice, another question, besides what body are we talking about, becomes what bodies to make? This is a question of ontological politics: 'a politics that has to do with the way in which problems are framed, bodies are shaped, and lives are pushed and pulled into one shape or another' (Mol, 2002: viii). In this more fluid idea of bodies, theory too can be seen as a body, which makes other bodies possible. As we have seen, *'theorizing, like experimenting, is a material practice*' (Barad, 2007: 55, original emphasis). But this is about more than theory as a critiquing (as opposed to critical) practice. Rather, it adds to the world. As Coleman and Ringrose point out, 'for Deleuze, concepts are not representative, reflective or descriptive but are creative' (2013: 7). Concepts do things! 'Theory is an inquiry, which is to say, a practice: a practice of the seemingly fictive world that empiricism describes; a study of the conditions of legitimacy of practices that is in fact our own' (Deleuze, 2001: 36).

The research questions posed above move from not only what realities are we talking about, but 'what realities to *make*?' (Law and Urry, 2004). Research becomes less about validity as truth and more to do with doing 'good' (Mol, 2002). But furthermore, it requires a different and more ethical style of thinking – away from judging, and towards 'caring' (Mol, 2014). It is this mode of caring that informed my research practice and, in this sense, took me away from doing my methodology 'properly' (see Law, 2004) to doing it 'with care'. As noted by Lury and Wakeford (2012), methods 'make a difference' or add to the world. This Deleuzian understanding resonates with Law and Urry's (2004) important paper 'Enacting the Social', which outlines the productive quality of social science. That is, in going against a separation of words and things in representational styles of thought, they make a case for the performativity of research that enacts social realities in practice. But, like Coleman and Ringrose (2013) have argued, for me, this is not about seeing social science as all powerful, 'rather, taking seriously the idea that methodology is a way of relating to multiply assembled worlds, suggests that social scientists are themselves entangled within the assemblages they seek to study' (2013: 6).

Therefore, drawing on Barad's (2003; 2007) 'agential realism', and in acknowledging these entanglements or assemblages, we must be aware of the 'cuts' that are being made in these productions of reality:

> The object of investigation is constructed through the enactment of particular cuts and not others. Which cuts are enacted are not a matter of choice in the liberal humanist sense; rather, the specificity of particular cuts is a matter of specific material practices through which the very notion of the human is differentially constituted.
>
> (Barad, 2007: 217)

In making her case, Barad draws on the human foetus not as a 'free-floating body located inside a technomaternal environment', but rather the result of 'particular historically and culturally specific intra-actions of material-discursive apparatuses' (2007: 217). What we know or rather 'relate to' is always part of these material-discursive constructions.

This book responds to the construction of injecting drug use as harmful. In this apparatus, 'harm' is created as 'independent, anterior, definite and singular' (Law, 2004: 36) as 'cuts' are made to the multiplicity of drug-using experiences and their effects (Dwyer and Moore, 2013; Pienaar et al., 2015). Refiguring these 'cuts', I have tried to change what Law (2004) calls the 'apparatus of reality production' to shift away from harm in 'detecting and amplifying' other bodies and affects. This attempts to respond to Law's assertion that 'there are a whole lot of realities that are not, so to speak, real, that would indeed have been so if the apparatus of reality production had been very slightly different' (2004: 33–4).

Therefore, to answer Law and Urry's (2004) question on 'what realities to make?' This book will attempt to produce better drug affects and ways of becoming-other with or without drugs based on a broader capacity to act. And, by attending care-fully to these practices, we can help bring them into being. A similar answer can be found in Fraser and Moore (2011)'s book, *Drug Effects*, which engages in an onto-epistemological understanding of cultural, medical and legal practices that, if reformulated, can produce better drug effects, and in Duff's (2014a) Deleuzian-informed concept of health, where health research and practice can contribute to increasing what a body can *do*. Through the methods laid out above, I will explore the usually unseen/said aspects of injecting drug use (in 'noticing bodies') which can do 'good' in a world where 'truth is no longer the final arbiter': 'In an ontological politics we might hope, instead, to interfere, to make some realities realer, others less so. The good of making a difference will live alongside – and sometimes displace – that of enacting truth' (Law, 2004, 67).

But beyond this idea of methods that 'make a difference', which focuses on enacted realities, my ethical commitments are also very much centred on a more ethical way of researching. Informed by a Deleuzian move away from Kantian judging more applicable to a world of validity and truth, that is, he says, 'the true dreamer is the one who goes out to verify something' (cited in Rajchman, 2000), I am taken with Fusco's (2008) conceptualisation of 'accurate' as something which is 'done with care'. In her discussion of how to research bodies, Fusco sought to 'make accurate comments about the everyday world', but not 'accurate' in a positivist sense of 'correct in all details', but rather in terms of the Latin word 'accuratus', which translates as 'done with care' (2008: 163). A thinking style of care was also taken up by Mol (2014) in a recent seminar in London in which she talked about 'caring' rather than 'explaining' or 'judging'. To paraphrase, she said that caring comes from inside, whereas to explain relies on an outside perspective. If something is 'done with care', it is not only done with a degree of efficiency, whatever that may be, but also done with compassion, import and empathy – this is not about grand representations, but about trying to relate *with* the world and care for it. This is most recently taken up by Maria Puig de la Bellacasa (2017) in her reworking of a feminist ethic of care for doing science and technology studies.

By mapping injecting bodies, I wish to attend to the neglected *affects*, *matter* and *practices*, in adding to the ways we know, experience and do bodies, *to do them better*. This is a diffractive approach that refuses *a priori* distinction between nature and culture: 'considering them together… means allowing any integral aspects to emerge (by not writing them out before we get started)' (Barad, 2007, 25). Each chapter in its own way disrupts binary thinking that has for too long constrained how we can think about drugs and our attachments to them, especially injecting, in mapping these be-comings and where they could be done better. Like Haraway's (2003; 2007) companion species, this is methodology of not just becoming-with but 'be-coming better': an enhancement beyond the individual (Latimer, 2013: 92). This is a venture that involves us all, in striving towards a 'common world' and politics.

Conclusion

A theoretical pursuit to register bodies as an ontologically flatter way of dealing with intra-acting entities in the injecting event is at the same time a methodological pursuit. As such, the methods described here move away from styles of representing bodies to 'detecting and amplifying' bodies and their collaborative forms. This requires paying attention to neglected bod-ies and 'things', and those forces or affects that also exceed them. Mapping bodies through drawing becomes an integral part of this move and an un-derstanding of bodies as always in flux, as they come to be affected and affect others in drug-using and -treatment events. My techniques of anal-ysis (unwittingly) aid these findings in enabling this flow and movement of bodies. It is in light of these bodies that resist categorisation that I reject an overly rigid form of coding and analysis. Therefore, rather than the meth-odological approach being prefigured, it is very much responsive to these injecting bodies as they interject and make themselves known. This inciden-tally leads towards a more intimately entangled or 'caring' style of research, where truth is usurped by good, and morality and judgement by ethics – an appealing idea that gets evoked throughout the book and fleshed out further in the conclusion.

Notes

1 For a more in-depth analysis of this shift, see Blackman (2008).
2 Although these terms can be used interchangeably, I have chosen to use 'socio-material' as I feel it accentuates the inseparability of the social and material.
3 See Dominguez Rubio (2016) on the discrepancy between things and objects and how things become objects.
4 See Jackson and Mazzei (2012) and MacLure (2013) for comprehensive critiques of coding.

Chapter 2

Thinking bodies

Conceptualising pleasure and not-so-pleasurable concepts

> We think and write for [drugs] themselves. We become [drug] so that the [drug] also becomes something else. The agony [or pleasure] of a [drug]... remains present in thought not through pity but as the zone of exchange between man and [drug] in which something of one passes into the other.
> Gilles Deleuze and Félix Guattari, 1994: 109

> As soon as I think about it [doing drugs], I have such mixed feelings about it, it's a really lovely feeling but my god the crap that comes with it.
> Lucy, 42 years old, injects heroin

Pleasure is hard to describe. As soon as Lucy starts to think about it, something else arrives. This sentence follows a discussion about the pleasures in which she gets overtaken by some of these feelings, rolling her eyes back to enact the extreme form of pleasure that emanates from her drug use, but then she jilts, flings her eyes wide open and says 'but as soon as I start thinking about it...'. There is something about 'thinking about it' that makes her uneasy. Drawing on Deleuze and Guattari's notion of doing philosophy as a kind of becoming-with the objects at stake, as a 'zone of exchange', I understand Lucy's difficulties in these conceptualisation practices as a form of embodied knowing. Concepts act in this space as much as bodies think. Concepts of addiction as antithetical to pleasure are immanent to the problem of enquiry. Through Lucy and other participants' accounts, it becomes clear that drugged pleasure is hard to conceptualise due to its antithetical yet paradoxical relationship to addiction, which means participants recognise pleasure in reference to autonomy, freedom and recreation, and deny pleasure in reference to compulsion, automaticity and dependency. Rather than analysing concepts as attempts to get closer to truths, subservient to life, which Deleuze and Guattari argue is often the case in sociology, here, I explore how they help to make the conditions for which life can be known and engaged (1994: 10).

By replacing the word 'animal' for 'drug' what I hope to suggest is that drugs too can become embedded in the bodies of people who use them as they become embedded with the drug, and it is through such intra-action that the conditions of thought are produced. Deleuze and Guattari use the figure of the animal in agony – 'a rat or the slaughter of a calf' – to suggest that, in thinking about the position of the animal, there is not simply a disconnected pity for the animal, but a connection at a very intimate level between the body of the animal and the thinker. 'This is the constitutive relationship of philosophy with nonphilosophy. Becoming is always double, and it is this double becoming that constitutes the people to come and the new earth' (Deleuze and Guattari, 1994: 109). What is possible is constituted through these relations. Agony, or as in this case pleasure, although I will get to agony, does not linger merely in a memory, in thought, in an emotion, but rather in the zones of exchange between the drug and the body. The drug has become part of the drug user like the drug user has become part of the drug, changing the conditions of thought and 'the people to come' in which 'something of one passes into the other' (Deleuze and Guattari, 1994: 109).

The conditions of thought and knowing have changed. Whether drug use can be conceptualised as pleasurable – how pleasure emerges in these conceptualisation practices – is contingent on these zones of exchange. The possibilities of thought are conditioned by these encounters, and likewise, these encounters are potentialised by the possibilities of what they can be thought to be. This becoming of bodies makes it hard to reflect on anything that has *been* previously as the conditions are always changing – the past is embedded in the future in a very literal way. What is made possible has changed, so as soon as Lucy starts to think about the pleasures of her drug use, other not-so-pleasurable concepts make themselves known. The agony does not get felt as a pity for oneself or a hatred for the drug, but as a stifling of the ability to think otherwise. 'The crap' that 'comes with' the drugs, as Lucy says, is difficult to think beyond. This is just one example of how the body has learnt to think *with* drugs and other drugged bodies.

Writing in relation to how scientists bond with the animals they study, Vinciane Despret uses the concept of 'embodied empathy' to account for how scientists' bodies are 'actively engaged' with the animals they observe. The conditions of what is knowable become embodied in these relationships. 'Embodied empathy' is 'a concept which describes feeling/seeing/thinking bodies that undo and redo each other, reciprocally though not symmetrically, as partial perspectives that attune themselves to each other' (Despret, 2013). By collapsing a false divide between the human and non-human, and the body and mind, in a dispersed sense of agency, the body can think (see also Savransky, 2016) and 'empathy is not experiencing with one's own body what the other experiences, but rather creating the possibilities of an embodied communication' (Despret, 2013: 51). The scientists' affinities with the animals they study and attempt to feel, see and think like are radically non-psychological as they become embodied and knowable through each another: 'scientists and animals are fleshy creatures which are enacted and enacting through their embodied choreography' (2013: 69).

In an earlier example of this embodied choreography, Despret (2004) draws on the historic accounts of Hans, 'the clever horse'. Hans learnt to answer complex mathematical questions correctly by attuning to the bodily signals of the person asking the questions. Bodies, in their attunement, or learning to become affected (Latour, 2004a), become able to think by embedding the conditions for action *with* the other body. The knowing or thinking self is only ever partial. As such, when pushed, participants in my study struggled deeply to *know* drugs and their feelings towards them. According to Haraway, 'the knowing self is partial in all its guises, never finished, whole, simply there and original; it is always constructed and stitched imperfectly' (cited in Despret, 2013: 61). This is seen here in participants' accounts of pleasure as they try to know something, a feeling or embodied part of the self, which is always on the move, always part of something else, other connections and affects, only ever in passing (Gomart and Hennion, 1999).

Following Latour, it is through this partiality of the knowing self that I have come to understand the antithetical relationship between pleasure and addiction as paradoxical in another way. Latour (1993) argues that the paradox of the moderns is that the more we try to separate, divide and dichotomise along cultural and natural, human and non-human lines, the more that hybridities will flourish. To take Lucy's opening sentence, the more she digs into the feelings of pleasure, the more intense 'the crap that comes with it' becomes until this is indeed what she is telling me about. The worlds of signs, subjects and concepts are not separate from but rather immanent to the world of things, objects and bodies. It is to this point that I turn first in this chapter, to where this paradoxical concept of pleasure as antithetical to addiction first made itself known. Second, I look at where such a concept may be coming from in the addiction sciences as a lack of freely chosen pleasure becomes a defining feature of addiction, but true to its construction, how it is both brought into being and collapsed by participants in their conceptualisations of pleasure (beyond subjective freedom). Third, I look at how pleasure has never been free, of the freely choosing and experiencing subject, but rather emergent from the bodies and concepts involved. In the last section, therefore, I come to think about pleasure as always in tension, caught up in social, discursive and material flows (Deleuze and Guattari, 1987; Latour, 1993). This makes knowing drugged pleasure in any singular way, divorced from the pains and harms of drug use, and by implication other embodied drug experiences, impossible as it is only ever in passing.

Conceptualising addicted pleasure: a modern paradox

> The more we forbid ourselves to conceive of hybrids, the more possible their interbreeding becomes – such is the paradox of the moderns.
>
> Bruno Latour, 1993: 12

Through my ethnographic observations and interviews with people who inject drugs and those who work with them, there was a strong sense that drug use was at points pleasurable, but it should not be, or rather, following the zones of exchange, could not be conceptualised in this way. Participants often spoke of the pleasures of their drug use, but then quickly followed this with a 'but' to indicate the many negative components. Participants would talk about their drug use, and pleasure would slip in, or participants would talk about pleasure, and addiction would force its way in. I choose these verbs carefully as participants' affective responses, when changing from *concepts* of pleasure to addiction, were often more sudden and intrusive. For example, in Lucy's account above, she starts to get upset when negative memories make themselves known, cutting her sentence off mid-flow. However, rather than viewing these positive and negative experiences as separate, pertaining either to memories of pleasure or addiction, they appeared to be in constant tension.

The antithetical relationship between addiction and pleasure revealed itself in many ways over the course of the project, not least in my own affective responses and sometimes debilitating fears around the contentiousness of the topic. I regularly asked myself why I was looking at pleasure in what was clearly – that is, in connection to the dominant discourses on addiction in the sciences, mass media and popular culture – a destructive and harmful phenomenon. If my own anxieties and affective responses were not enough to go off in noticing how stabilised an antithetical dynamic of pleasure/addiction had become, this realisation was soon reached early on in my research when I visited one of the drug treatment organisations to speak to the manager and a group of service users from the regional service user committee to seek their feedback, and as part of the governance of research, to gain approval for the study to go ahead.

Meeting with the manager in his office, he was enthusiastic about the project, but concerned that I might have misjudged the service user group. He told me that my project's interest in drugs' pleasures might be more relevant to young people who liked to sit around getting 'stoned' on cannabis rather than to people who were injecting heroin on a daily basis 'out of an addiction'. In this, he was pointing to the differences between recreational and dependent drug use. After talking to the manager about these issues and trying to explain why it might be relevant, I was invited downstairs to meet with and present my proposal to the regional service user committee. The twelve members, who were seated around a large boardroom table, had read the research proposal in advance. The manager again raised his concerns, saying that my project aims sounded more akin to cannabis use than heroin or crack cocaine use, and this was discussed amongst the group. On the back foot, I reinstated that this was just one aspect of the research and I was not going to push it if people saw it as inapplicable. The Chair, who described himself as a recovering heroin addict, talked about how he did not know anyone who would see their drug use as pleasurable, and if they did, it was just a 'superficial' aspect, and used as a mechanism for 'denying' the more underlying issues. In this sense, pleasure was not a legitimate concern, or as a concern, it was only worth exploring in terms of what it was deemed to be 'covering up'. This sparked a long discussion about the harms that drug use had caused the members of the group and other people they knew.

It seemed that pleasure was just not that relevant, that is, until one man, sitting across from me, and waiting for a moment's silence, interrupted and said that, as soon as I started talking about injecting, a 'pleasurable sensation', what he described as a 'tingling', took place at his old injection site. Suddenly, much to people's surprise, including the man himself, pleasure had entered the room. His body had spoken, it had, to use Magdalena Harris's (2009; 2015) vocabulary, awoken a 'latent desire', a visceral response that reappears at unsuspecting moments. Although the man went on to recount some of the difficulties (e.g. living in a crack house) and tiresomeness of being in 'full blown addiction', his body, in that moment, thinking with the drug and other drugged bodies (e.g. syringe), enacted pleasure, and pulling away from the group and their current discourses, he spoke about the excitement of those days. In this account, memories and thoughts of pleasure were not located in the mind, nor conjured up through the body, but rather, had always been there in these embodied zones of exchange with the body, lying low until stirred.

I was taken aback by this man's response, and his embodied support for the relevance of pleasure. This was a brave move as bodies regularly get shut out and ignored in drug treatment services and research (Harris, 2015). It was also clear this was going to be no exception, with others in the group already showing their distaste towards embodied feelings and notably pleasure, which was seen to mask the dysfunctional reward system and destruction addiction causes. And, indeed, his response was moved on from quickly. Pleasure undoubtedly occupied a difficult space that needed to be carefully managed.

Making concepts: keeping pleasure and addiction apart

Approaching bodies as sociomaterial processes, I want to think about how concepts also act in conceptualisation practices. I look here at how a concept of addiction is made in opposition to pleasure, moreover, how a lack of pleasure is a defining feature of addiction, and how such concepts make their way into participants' accounts of pleasure (or a lack of it). Proponents of the incentive-sensitisation theory of addiction divide drug use between 'liking' and 'wanting'. The work of Kent Berridge has been particularly influential in establishing this divide. Addiction, according to this theory, is a reward-system dysfunction: 'The incentive-sensitization theory posits the essence of drug addiction to be excessive amplification specifically of psychological "wanting", especially triggered by cues, without necessarily an amplification of "liking'"(Berridge and Robinson, 2016: 670).

Although 'wanting' and 'liking' can be linked, they are said to reside in separate parts of the brain and function independently: 'wanting' is seen as 'incentive salience', whilst 'liking' is seen as 'subjective pleasure'. In terms of this 'wanting' or what they call 'objective' pleasure, 'rewards may influence behaviour even in the absence of being consciously aware of them' (Berridge et al., 2010). In other words, 'wanting' is a matter of automaticity, that is, 'objectively' known (e.g. through positron emission tomography [PET] scans), beyond conscious awareness, whilst 'liking' is said to be 'subjectively' and consciously known and governed. They depict how, over the course of using drugs, the relationship between 'liking' and 'wanting' changes, with 'wanting' increasing and 'liking' decreasing as the drug use moves from 'casual' to 'compulsive': 'The transition from casual drug use to compulsive addiction is posited to be owing to drug-induced sensitization of mesocorticolimbic mechanisms of incentive salience ["wanting"]' (2010: 16).

As 'addiction' progresses, 'liking', or 'subjective pleasure', is said to diminish. This is summed up in another paper by Robinson and Berridge: 'we suggest that drug pleasure becomes less and less important during the transition to addiction' (2003: 46). The lack of freely chosen pleasure, therefore, becomes a defining feature of addiction as a brain disease. This is evident in the flourishing area of research on 'craving' as a phenomenon of the 'dysfunctional' reward system, which is again isolated from 'subjective' pleasure. An editorial special of the prominent science journal, *Nature*, epitomises this deficit position:

> Drug addiction is a disease. Images of the brains of addicts show alterations in regions crucial to learning and memory, judgement and decision-making, and behavioural control. Drugs imitate natural neurotransmitters, resulting in false or abnormal messages being sent around neural circuits. *The brain's central reward system is overstimulated and flooded with dopamine.* The brain adapts to this flood by turning down its ability to respond to dopamine – so addicts take more and more of the drug to push dopamine levels higher. Changes in other *reward-system* neurotransmitters such as glutamate can *impair cognitive function.* And the triggering of subconscious memory systems leads to conditioning, so environmental cues such as particular people or places set off *uncontrollable cravings.* None of that is particularly controversial, at least among scientists.
>
> (*Nature* editorial, 2014, my emphases)

Instead of 'subjective' pleasure, there is an 'overstimulated' reward system, leading to 'impaired cognitive function' and 'uncontrollable cravings'.

Therefore, to return to our unexpected encounter with pleasure in the service user committee above, an embodied pleasure had entered where it supposedly does not belong. As such, it was carefully managed, and even I did not know how to respond. Besides acknowledging his feeling, I was at a loss with what to say (a reaction not dissimilar to a service provider, Matt's account below when pleasure entered his servicer user group). There was an uneasiness about the atmosphere, which perhaps reaffirms on an affective level the strength of this antithetical dynamic between pleasure and addiction. But this is by no means a 'natural' distinction, as the situation also highlights the proactive work being done to keep pleasure and addiction apart – the freely chosen pleasure of the social cannabis use, away from the addictive misinformed pleasure of heroin or crack cocaine use, that is, we are told, 'pleasure' cannot really exist beyond 'denial' for those using drugs in a dependent way. However, ironically, these very practices of maintaining the divide are what expose its fallacy.

From a critical sociological perspective, the importance of maintaining this divide between addiction and pleasure could be seen in terms of what O'Malley and Valverde (2004) have identified as a link between discourses of pleasure and freedom in the governance of drug users. In their paper, *Pleasure, Freedom and Drugs*, O'Malley and Valverde trace how pleasure since the eighteenth century has been linked to discourses of reason and freedom (i.e. 'liking' or 'subjective pleasure'), 'so that problematic drug consumption appears both without reason (e.g. "bestial") and unfree (e.g. "compulsive"), and thus not as "pleasant"' (2004: 25). They argue that this is made possible through shifts in governance which mean:

> Pleasure, especially as in the figure of the felicity calculus, is at the heart of liberal constructions of the rational and free subject. Pleasure and rationality are foundationally linked, precisely because the pleasure/ pain couple is a given in the liberal constitution of rational calculation.
> (O'Malley and Valverde, 2004: 28)

A concept of pleasure as freely chosen is central to governmentality in 'advanced liberal' societies like the UK, which are said to operate paradoxically *through freedom*. Nikolas Rose has written extensively on the matter and explores various ways that freedom is used in contemporary society to produce particular types of governable citizens. This work is summed up in a collaborative piece by Rose, O'Malley and Valverde:

> [...] central to contemporary strategies for governing the soul was the creation of freedom. Subjects were obliged to be free and were required to conduct themselves responsibly, to account for their own lives and their vicissitudes in terms of their freedom. Freedom was not opposed to government. On the contrary, freedom, as choice, autonomy,

self-responsibility, and the obligation to maximize one's life as a kind of enterprise, was one of the principal strategies of what Rose termed advanced liberal government.

(Rose et al., 2006: 90–91)

Neoliberal pleasure is intrinsically tied up with notions of freedom, rationality and reason. It is within this framework that certain kinds of drug use is seen to be without 'freedom', without 'rationality', and consequently without 'pleasure' (O'Malley and Valverde, 2004). This chimes with Eve Sedgwick's observation that 'the object of addiction has become precisely enjoyment of "the ability to choose freely, and freely choose health"' (1993: 132). By this, she means, 'addiction' has proliferated as the polar opposite of 'free choice' – 'so long as "free will" has been hypostatised... for just so long has a hypostatitised "compulsion" had to be available as a counterstructure always internal to it' (1993: 134). Consequently, pleasure (as free) and addiction (as compulsion) emerge as one.

In this mode of thought, the lack of freely chosen pleasure (or 'liking') is central to the governance of drug users as lacking 'free choice'. Therefore, drug users 'are problematic [and in need of controlling] because they throw into question the very presuppositions of moral consciousness, self-control and self-advancement through legitimate consumption upon which governmental regimes of freedom depend' (Rose, 2000: 321).

For O'Malley (2002), this governance extends beyond the epidemic of 'free will' captured in Sedgwick's analysis. He also sees a 'governance through freedom' in relation to, at the time, a newly formed public health programme of 'harm minimisation', in which drug users or addicts (once seen as the inverse of rationality and reason) are produced as rational health-choosing subjects: 'ironically then, the dilemmas of freedom and constraint that for so long haunted the governance of drugs have not gone away... Rather, they have assumed new guises' (2002: 294).

Although, for me, freedom seemed to be existing in a different way, and thus, these are the wrong dilemmas, I will stay with this line of thinking for a little longer in order to make my argument. To do so, an important link is missing. This is the assumed distinction between 'recreational' and 'addictive' drug use, which remains unchallenged. For example, in O'Malley and Valverde's (2004) paper, they uncritically direct their attention to 'problematic drug use'. One might have thought this construct to be critiqued in their comparison of Hogarth's 'beer street' and 'gin lane' – the former representing alcohol consumption as virtuous and the latter as vice – but it remained foreclosed. This distinction that continues to proliferate in social scientific thought and drug policy and practice is, for me, one that stands at the centre of such governance (what I am calling it for now). That is, addictive drug use falls neatly into a category of 'wanting', whilst recreational drug use falls neatly into a category of 'liking'. By the social sciences speaking to these divides rather than against or across them, the dichotomies remain.[1] What I am suggesting is that, without much awareness, these categories get remade in studies that otherwise try to challenge them. This means that pleasure continues to be very hard to discuss in relation to 'addictive' drug use[2] and causes participants all kinds of trouble as they try to make these separations. Therefore, in asking participants to reflect on pleasure in the interviews, I inadvertently imported a concept of pleasure as freely chosen, which meant pleasure often got denied in light of addiction or compulsion and accepted in recourse to subjective freedom. Malik, who was in his 40s and experiencing a strained relationship with drugs in which he said he both wanted to and didn't want to inject 'speedballs' [a combination of heroin and crack cocaine], says:

> Pleasure does come into it, it did come into it, but I tell you now, for the last 3 years of so, no, it has not been pleasurable. There's the *obsession* in me to use anyway, cos I've done it for so long, I will obsess over it. And *my brain* will make these lovely, I'll remember the good bits.

Pleasure is existing in light of a certain freedom, so that without this perceived freedom, there is no pleasure, it has been overtaken by an 'obsession' in the 'brain'.

On the flip side, a presence of pleasure was often confirmed in relation to a concept of subjective freedom. Mike and Paula, for example, validate their drugged pleasures through several contrasts to addiction (as compulsion), including 'recreational'/'habitual', 'cravings'/'want', 'want to'/'need to', 'quick buzz'/'having to', 'pleasure'/'need' and 'able to say no'/not able to say no:

> Yeah, *it's more recreational now than habitual.* And for once it feels good to be able to have money and know that you can do it if you want to do it. If you don't want to do it, it's fine. I sit there and think to myself, I don't get many cravings these days, thank god, but when I do, when I do think about it sometimes, or if someone mentions it, and I think well I haven't used for 5 days or over a week, you know, so why do it now, so I'm not easily lead into it, I'll only do it when I want to do or when I feel I need to do it. It is more for just like a quick buzz, a quick euphoria, *to have a good time, rather than like having to do it.*
>
> (Mike, 34 years old, injects 'speedballs')

> It's *pleasure more than need now.* And I can say no, I never used to be able to say no, that word never used to come out of my mouth, so I've actually learnt the word, to say 'no, I'm not doing it'.
>
> (Paula, 60 years old, injects heroin)

Even though all the study participants, if seeking treatment, would meet the *DSM-V* (American Psychiatric Association, 2013) criteria for an 'addictive disorder', they often drew on the dichotomy between recreational and addictive drug use and these 'different levels' to distinguish their practice as pleasure-seeking and within their control, and thus not addictive. Ajay, who injects 'speedballs', says:

> It can be habitual, it depends how strong your soul is, like if you choose to be a waster, like obviously you've seen wasters, you've obviously done other interviews with other people, and obviously their body doesn't look well, they don't eat properly. There's *different levels* [pause], *I use because I want to use, not because I'm a street junkie, I use because I enjoy using.*

Vargas (2010) cautions us against asking why people use drugs due to the susceptibility of pathologised responses – 'it's not enough to ask "why do people use drugs?" and "what is the meaning of drugs?", which is seen to lead to answers usually premised on "error", "lack" or "weakness"' (2010: 210). I would add to this a warning about how pleasure, which, existing in opposition to a dysfunctional 'wanting', also, conversely, reproduces such pathologies and stigmatising identities. Ajay refers to a 'strength of soul', which is lacking in 'street junkies'. Therefore, following Duff (2014a), I have come to conclude that I was asking too much:

> the trouble with conventional approaches to drug use is that they ask rather too much of the drug user. The user bears responsibility for most of the dynamics of consumption, and subsequently remains culpable for any of the harm [but also pleasure] generated therein.
>
> (2014a: 142–3)

I was asking participants to reflect on something they were not entirely in control of. That is, as we have seen, thinking is conditioned by the 'zones of exchange' between bodies, where concepts too can act and become something new. It is perhaps not that surprising then that just as easily as a concept of pleasure-as-free came into being, it started to fall away and become something else. That is, to follow Latour's (1993) modern paradox, the more we try to make separations between pleasure and addiction, freedom and compulsion, subjectivity and objectivity, the mind and body, and the conceptual and real, the more we generate hybrids. Following both Vargas's (2010) use of Gabriel Tarde and Duff's (2014a) use of Gilles Deleuze, pleasure is not stable, but a matter of the event, which is anything but freely chosen. In reifying the subject through asking about pleasure, particular conditions are borne out. Of interest here is namely a dichotomy between pleasure and addiction. But in letting the human subject go, and attuning to or 'noticing' (Stewart, 2007) what was brought up in other less directed parts of the interview, where the subject was not so prominent (authoritative or agentic), these dichotomous ways of thinking and doing drugs, such as 'liking' versus 'wanting', could unfold and become known as something else.

Some participants conversely talked about their 'addictive' drug use in terms of pleasure, in which, going against the pleasure/addiction dichotomy, they continued using drugs because of the pleasures. For example, talking about her recent shift to heroin injecting from smoking, Gwen, a woman in her early fifties, says 'actually I'm stoned, this is nice, so it's a bit addictive in that way, you want to do it again'. 'Speedballing', for most participants, was felt to be particularly enjoyable and addictive: 'As soon as I started doing the speedball, *I like it so much*, but it makes me do *one after the other after the other*' (Grigor, twenty-nine years old). Even more defiantly, 'the addict' was seen as a discerning pleasure seeker. Mike says: 'Well, the addict inside me is happy, because I'm getting a good bit of thing [crack] for once'. The addict, in this case, has taste. And some of Mike's more dangerous decisions were also taken out of pleasure rather than 'need':

> I mean when I first did my groin *I didn't need to*, I weren't in a situation where I had no veins left, I did, but, again, my friend was doing it and you know, I said what's the difference and he said 'oh yeah, it hits you harder, its stronger, and hits you so much quicker'.

A similar sense of pleasure-seeking, rather than necessity or 'need', can be seen in Meg's account of neck injecting:

MEG: I have used my feet and I have used my neck, I've never used my groin ever.

FD: Was your neck because you couldn't find... [she pre-empted that I was going to say a vein]

MEG: No, it wasn't that, someone said oh you get a *better hit*, it goes straight to your head, and they did it for me, I didn't do it on my own... It does go to your head quicker, I suppose because it's nearer your brain.

Trying to make sense of the antithetical dynamic of pleasure/addiction, as both brought into being and collapsed by participants, I am unconvinced that a theory of governmentality goes far enough to understand the extent of the difficulties participants faced in discussing the pleasures of injecting drug use. In privileging addiction as a matter of discourse (used to control certain drugged pleasures), governmentality theories tend to underplay the materiality of injecting, which both neglects some aspects of the drug assemblage (beyond concepts) and the somatic feelings enacted. For instance, Sedgwick says:

> The locus of addictiveness cannot be the substance itself and can scarcely even be the body itself, but must be some overarching abstraction that governs the narrative relations between them.
>
> (1993: 131)

Furthermore, for Bunton and Coveney, these abstract tendencies are seen in relation to the wider dichotomous make-up of the drug field which has been neatly divided between the disciplines:

> Psychology and neurophysiology have developed biological foundations for emotions, including pleasure, as an inherently human phenomenon. Central neurological pathways are credited with the passage of pleasure-receiving signals, and specific parts of the brain have been identified as centres where pleasure is registered (Warburton, 1994). By contrast, sociologists have situated pleasures in time, space and specific discourses seeing pleasure as a socio-cultural construction.
>
> (2011: 11)

From becoming-with injecting bodies in this research, there are clear inadequacies in both the discursive and biological models, as both fail to cope with the complexities of pleasure and addiction, mind and body and human and non-human as already entangled. This has encouraged me to think about the concept of freedom and pleasure as freely chosen in another way. Rather than understanding freedom in the neoliberal sense – as a paradox based on 'governance through freedom' – I have come to consider freedom through a distinctly 'modern' paradox (Latour, 1993). In Latour's seminal text, *We Have Never Been Modern*, he explains how we have never made the separations between nature and culture that in 'western' societies we so unrelentingly follow. Where postmodern theories have tried to eradicate such binaries in recourse to social or discursive construction, Latour argues that such divides have rather never existed. Therefore, even though the 'Modern Constitution', as seen here in the addiction sciences, works tirelessly to *make* pleasure seem freely chosen (of the subject), and so *pleasure can be addictive but addiction cannot be pleasurable*, participants' conceptualisations indicate something else. For Latour, what makes this a modern paradox is not its capacity to govern through freedom but that the more we try to make these separations, the more the complexities seem to proliferate. Furthermore, and to be developed in Chapter 4, as participants work to keep themselves within their subject boundaries (that refuse drugs' pleasures), harmful conflicts can emerge. Next, however, I turn to this paradox that seems to get realised as participants, under my invitation, try to *think about* their drug use. It is under these thinking conditions in which they try to separate pleasure from pain, choice from autonomy and the empirical from the conceptual, that these tensions make themselves known and it becomes apparent that such separations are impossible for they have never been there.

Pleasure has never been free: 'As soon as I start to think about it…'

> Here on the left, are the things themselves; there, on the right, is the *free* society of speaking, *thinking subjects*, values and signs. Everything happens in the middle, everything passes between the two, everything happens by way of mediation, translation and networks, but this space does not exist, it has no place. It is unthinkable, *the unconscious of the moderns*.
>
> Bruno Latour, 1993: 37, my emphasis

Above, we have seen how addiction sciences work to separate subjective 'liking' from objective 'wanting' – or what I have come to think about as keeping pleasure 'free', of the free choosing subject. But, drawing on Deleuze and Guattari, and Latour, such separations have never existed. In this section, I will consider how such a realisation emerges in participants' accounts. In this sense, 'addicts' once again get 'too close' to the paradox, but, where for Rose (2000) they have got too close to the empty ideal of 'freedom', or for Bjerg (2008), for example, they have 'got too close to the body', for me, they have got too close to the 'nonhuman' or, more accurately, the even more problematic more-than-human. As Haraway says: 'Cyborg unities are monstrous and illegitimate; in our present political circumstances, we could hardly hope for more potent myths for resistance and recoupling' (1991a: 154). These intense human-non-human relationships threaten to jostle the 'modern' fallacy that pleasure and other sociomaterial feelings can be split between nature/culture, human/non-human, mind/body, empirical/conceptual, etc.

Therefore, in this study, I am trying to get people to think about the unthinkable – 'the unconscious of the moderns' – the networks, or, the 'zones of exchange' (Deleuze and Guattari, 1994). Answering questions about drugs' pleasures was invariably hard for participants, especially when it came to the very issue of why it was such a difficult matter to discuss (as it would require awareness of these constructions). Indeed, at times I decided not to even ask about pleasure (for reasons that were unbeknown at the time, other than the feeling that asking about pleasure in relation to addictive drug use was inappropriate). In a similar way to what happened in the regional service use committee when pleasure entered, this uncertainty around how to respond to pleasure was further illustrated in a service provider, Matt's recollection of its uncomfortable entry into a group he runs for people preparing to access residential detoxification and rehabilitation.

Pleasure is not supposed to be there, but by being there, it starts to expose the pleasure/addiction binary as a fallacy and thus the networks that bring it into being.

I asked, referring to his previous role as a key worker: 'So can I ask you, in your key working sessions, did pleasure ever come up in relation to people's drug use?' Matt replies: 'It did'. Pushing him further, I asked: 'And how did you, like, respond to that?' And he then explains more about this difficult situation, for reasons he still does not fully understand. I will quote his reply in full to give an impression of the level of confusion and difficulty that pleasure arouses.

> Well it's a difficult one to deal with. Not only in key-working sessions but actually in the last detox group that I had last Thursday this very thing came up. This client came up and he was very, very clear that he wanted to change and he wanted to stop using but he enjoyed the use of heroin so much that he was going to find it very difficult to live without it, and *he kept saying that.* Now the way I *dealt with* that, well, *it's very difficult* because we've all experienced that in our transition, all of us have enjoyed using something at some point, that's why we started, nobody would have used and not experienced any form of pleasure otherwise it wouldn't have gone any further. *It's a difficult one to deal with,* I've got to say that it's not one that has come up very often. At a drug service, I would say the vast majority of individuals, when they are presenting for treatment, then they're asking for, certainly substitute medication, have forgotten how it was to enjoy their use and they're only using to stop withdrawing and so it hasn't really come up that often, so it hasn't really been addressed that often. When it does come up, I have to admit that *I'm at a little bit of a loss to know how to deal with it, it's not an easy one to deal with, but for sure, it's there,* and it's completely understandable of course. Some substances are extremely moreish, it's, you know, it's what's called positive reinforcement, you know, you take a substance, you feel better, you feel good I should say. So but, I'd say, it's not something that comes up too much.

Matt explains that pleasure rarely comes up, but when it does, it can be 'difficult to deal with', that is, to make sense of or explain away in light of an addiction which disallows pleasure. Note how the term 'deal with' is used four times in this excerpt, a feeling of pleasure cannot just be, but has to be dealt with. This is particularly stark in a treatment setting where workers are trained to actively challenge 'ambivalence',[3] which could prevent or derail recovery. To revisit the example I mentioned in the Introduction, one service user I assessed for treatment claimed her reason for injecting heroin and taking other drugs was for enjoyment – on asking her 'reasons for drug use' she resolutely said 'for fun' – but when her key-worker joined us, the worker was quick to refute this answer and instead link her drug use back to a miscarriage. A recourse to pleasure, in this environment, was felt to be inappropriate and needed to be rethought. The worker explained to me that if the service user was not willing to concede, she may not be serious about recovery, and may have wanted substitute medication for a different purpose, like stabilising or managing her current drug use, which, as I will explain in Chapter 5, has become an increasingly unacceptable way to engage in drug treatment. Thinking about this experience in my questions posed to Matt, I was keen to understand these difficulties around pleasure further. I asked: 'And I suppose there's a fear that if you spend too much time talking about the positive then they might...?' However, this comment unexpectedly prompted a new line of thought, and Matt enthusiastically interjects with a jolted recollection:

> Yeah, you've got to be careful. *But*, the vast majority of people that I access are experiencing moderate to profound depression, mild to moderate suicide ideation, at the very least. Some, a lot of my clients, I've done two clients at the moment in rehab whose self-harming has really reached a peak, with admissions to hospital under Section of the Mental Health Act so it's as far removed from pleasure as you can get. That is my general feeling of the clients that we deal with, they're really not experiencing very much pleasure, *or at least they are not letting us know*, they certainly... Maybe it's because we don't talk about it... They may think, the role that they're *playing as client*, they may feel that it's not appropriate to discuss pleasure. I was quite surprised last week when the client in the group did start talking about it.

Here, Matt comes to question the absence of pleasure in light of these concepts of 'depression', 'suicidal ideation' and 'self-harm', which are 'as far removed from pleasure as you can get' and very much in-keeping with the addiction he is concerned about (and perhaps what leads him to being a bit perturbed by my line of enquiry). But more than this, coming back on himself, he also understands pleasure's absence in relation to its social position, that is, the performative aspect of how pleasure and addiction are kept apart: 'they're really not experiencing very much pleasure, *or at least they are not letting us know*'. He talks about a 'client role' in which pleasure is an inappropriate topic for discussion. The antithetical dynamic between pleasure/addiction starts to show cracks, and the paradox (pleasure can be addictive but addiction cannot be pleasurable) begins to become exposed, but perhaps not in the way we might expect. What if Matt was being kind to me? For instance, in hindsight, it seems that he was only ever tentatively offering me this second explanation:

> Or, *at least* they are not letting us know... *Maybe* it's because we don't talk about it... They *may* think, the role that they're playing as client, they *may* feel that it's not appropriate to discuss pleasure.

What if, instead, I try to take his initial response seriously, and in many cases, pleasure does not actually exist for his clients: 'That is my general feeling of the clients that we deal with, they're really not experiencing very much pleasure'. In fact, Matt's response reminds me of Latour's (1993) point in relation to the confusing status of science studies, and, as such, commentators 'turn it into nature, politics or discourse'. Latour explains how everything gets drawn up into these categories of 'nature' or 'culture', and so I wonder whether this was what was happening when I questioned the existence of pleasure. Perhaps I unwittingly encouraged Matt to make these 'cultural' or 'social' interpretations. In view of an ontological politics, it no longer feels so contradictory that in the treatment centre (as opposed to some accounts given in the interviews) pleasure does not exist. For those two clients who had to be admitted to hospital for self-harm under the Mental Health Act, they are connecting-up not only with concepts of addiction, but other medical and legal concepts and bodies in which it is hardly surprising that pleasure has seized to exist.

This is more than an understanding of different contexts requiring different 'roles' (e.g. hiding pleasure to conform to drug services that may rely on a concept of addiction without pleasure), but rather the context is producing different conditions for thought (or zones of exchange). The interview set-up and researcher are also in no doubt part of this. But to take an interest in these materialities is not to say that a lack of pleasure is given (like with the addiction model of objective 'wanting'). Indeed, following Mol, ontology is 'brought into being, sustained, or allowed to wither away in common, day-to-day, sociomaterial practices' (2002: 6). As I have shown, there are several such practices in both drug research and services that try to keep pleasure as 'free', separate from and antithetical to 'addictive' wants. This is not given, but proactively maintained, for example, the man who spoke of a pleasurable sensation at the regional service user committee and the woman who said she used drugs for fun were both quickly redirected towards more negative feelings of pain and suffering. To take seriously an absence of pleasure is not to suggest that service users are simply playing a role, as a form of social conditioning or way of learning how to access services, or, indeed, that it is due to a shift in neurotransmitters from 'liking' to 'wanting', but actively 'absented' (Law, 2004) through sociomaterial networks, and hence why it has to be 'dealt with'. Pleasure in this context risks disrupting and thus exposing the construction of addiction as antithetical to pleasure.

Continuing with this argument, it is interesting that Matt highlights the drug service as a pivotal space-time in this movement of service users' experiences from pleasure to harm:

> At a *drug service*, I would say the vast majority of individuals, when they are *presenting for treatment*, and those that are asking for, certainly

substitute medication, have forgotten how it was to enjoy their use and they're only using to stop withdrawing.

Matt's account is quite different to many of the people who inject drugs that I interviewed, but in exploring it further, it starts to make sense. Let's imagine being a potential client, entering this drug service for the first time, as Matt says, 'presenting for treatment' and asking for substitute medication. First you would be met with a tall, encroaching building tucked around a corner, down a side alley; there is an anonymous door with a 'please buzz for entry' sign. On being let in, there is a loud release of the hinge which exaggerates the door's size and weight, the staircase is dimly light and there are two sets of stairs with a turn in the middle which means at first you are climbing towards a blank wall. You will then reach the receptionist who sits behind a glass shutter with a small opening to speak through. After the receptionist has made sure you have an appointment or there is an available duty worker, you are signed in and buzzed through to the waiting area. Through a maze of doors (which took me months to navigate), a large space opens up, with a wall mounted television playing daytime TV, usually chat shows, on mute, three-tiered faux-leather sofas, and posters that line the walls with messages and service information about recovery and drug-related health problems. Off this central space are two small 'session rooms' housing a desk and an old desktop computer, with splayed out leaflets and oral swabs for drug testing. This description is not to criticise the organisation or the staff who often did their best to make the environment as inviting as possible, but to think through what Matt's statement might mean, ontologically.[4] That is, it is in no doubt in my mind, to twist Matt's meaning slightly, that most people arriving at the drug service in this somewhat bleak and clinical environment 'presenting for treatment' *had* 'forgotten how it was to enjoy their use'.

Unlike an epistemological understanding of politics, where discourses produce ways of knowing (in line with a governmentality understanding of freedom), an ontological politics questions the stability of our very being (Mol, 1999). Following this lead, a lack of pleasure is more than 'performative'; rather, it is produced and embodied through a network of bodies, things and concepts. However, some realities are more possible than others as material environments afford certain ways of being. This often meant there was a tension between pleasure and the social pains/consequences of taking drugs as pleasure got articulated in the service. Bodies, plugged into these different networks, and thus potentialised in both directions, were only ever partially constituted. Participants tried to separate the immediate feelings from the longer term, the bodily from the social, but they would not hold. In fact, but in Latour's terms to be expected, the more participants tried to distinguish the (somatic and social) pleasures from the pains, the more the interbreeding seemed to occur.

Pleasure-in-tension: '… It's a really lovely feeling but my god the crap that comes with it'

In the chapter so far, I have drawn attention to how addiction/pleasure gets made as antithetical in addiction sciences and the drug service, but, testimony to its modern construction, how it also gets complicated in participant accounts. Whether pleasure exists for people to talk about is neither natural (given) nor cultural (performative), but a product of networks or 'zones of exchange', to use Deleuze and Guattari's term. I will now look further at how these complexities manifest in two accounts from Lucy and Ajay, who, in their different ways, encapsulate these tensions. As they moved through networks of bodies, discourses, things and forces, new conditions for thought emerged in which 'the crap' or 'the agony' (Deleuze and Guattari, 1994: 109), which until this point had been forgotten about, resurfaces, for this is not about having 'pity' or distaste for drugs and drugged bodies, but having a connection on an embodied level with drugs, in which drugs have become part of the body. In talking about pleasure, Lucy and Ajay tried to separate out pleasure from other drug 'effects' or affects, but, true to its modern constitution, this was not possible, and the complexity or 'crap' just multiplied. This brings about a tension in which talking about pleasure in this context of addictive drug use becomes very hard, not necessarily because it does not exist (chemically) or does not belong (in a governmentality sense), but because concepts of addiction are always ready to act or rather have already acted in making the conditions that are possible for thought. Pleasure is literally in tension in these zones of exchange as bodies become-with drugs and their assemblages – drugged pleasure is only ever a partial affinity (Despret, 2013).

I will now quote Lucy's words in full, as the vibrancy of the account would be lost if paraphrased.

LUCY: …But then I *slipped* back into gear because it was, it's a really weird mistress, or whatever they say, you just think you can leave it and I hope to beat it one day, but it's something that unfortunately it does do what it says. It does wrap you up in cotton wool.

FD: Can you tell me a bit more about these feelings?

LUCY: Well the first time I took it, it is orgasmic, I felt like I was floating on the bed. Like, it was, because he started before me, he [her partner] was quite cross, 'you've got that first feeling', and getting really jealous. And I thought 'oh my god' (rolling her eyes back, suggesting an overwhelming pleasure)… *but I don't want to advertise it*, I'm just saying… but that's what you're *chasing*. But then, when it comes to, what's so *dangerous* about it, it's weird because my sister was very good at the beginning because she had a boyfriend who was very much into heroin and she was so scared for me, she was like please don't go into that extent, and of course you lie to people and say 'oh I'm not', but I was holding down jobs and (stops suddenly). *But even though I keep talking about the good side of it, I have such* (starts to stutter/quiver), *as soon as I think about it, I have such mixed feelings about it, it's a really lovely feeling but my god the crap that comes with it,* the stress of getting the money, going to the (cuts off), hiding the secret, taking something, having a hit in the toilet, not having gear, going home dripping, trying to hold down a job where you're hallucinating because you're withdrawing and pouring with sweat, and someone saying can you fax this and you're just thinking I want to go, I want to go, but once you're comfortable at home and you've got all your paraphernalia, it's lovely.

To reiterate, Lucy says, *'as soon as I start thinking about it, I have such mixed feelings, it's a really lovely feeling but my god the crap that comes with it'*. She then elaborates on some of this 'crap'. For me, this highlights the difficulties participants found in separating out not only the more immediate feelings from the more lasting, the bodily from the social, but also, more importantly for this chapter, the experiential or real from the conceptual. This is not because they are separate, but precisely because they emanate together. There is something in the thinking itself which puts pleasure in tension – 'as soon as I start thinking about it' – in which it is attached to social stigma, painful withdrawals, financial difficulties, etc. In this sense, as already argued, concepts are more than a way of describing worlds, subservient to life, whilst thinking is an effect of external forces as much as internal ones. Therefore, to understand how pleasure is thought about as always in tension, I wish to attend to the networks in Lucy and Ajay's accounts that produce these thoughts, and thus what this could say more widely about how drugged pleasures come to be conceptualised in research, practice and policymaking, and how this could enable alternative, more productive concepts for thinking and doing drugs.

For Lucy, as she describes above, it is in being caught up with networks of physical dependency, changing family dynamics and negative social attitudes that things become 'dangerous'. More specifically, it is in lying to her family, 'hiding the secret [of using]', 'the stress of getting the money', 'having a hit in the toilet', 'withdrawing and pouring with sweat' and 'trying to hold down a job'. I find the role of sweat, the toilet and the fax machine to be particularly prominent and powerful actors. There are discourses connected to the toilet which means having to use it for anything other than its purpose is highly stigmatised. Sweating is attached to a particularly gendered discourse of shame. And the fax machine affords an office (and, I would suggest, gendered) professionalism and servitude that she is struggling to conform to. But once Lucy is at home with her *'paraphernalia, it's lovely'*. As these networks change, Lucy's feelings towards her injecting change and as she reflects, they begin to overlap and merge. To reinforce Mol's sentiment, 'as actors come to participate in different "networks", discourses, logics, modes of ordering, practices, things get complex' (2010: 260). Lucy tries to separate (in line with the Modern Constitution) herself from the drugs, thought from the world, past from the present, and the bodily from the social, but this is not possible and causes tension. To revisit Latour and Deleuze and Guattari, everything is at once material, social and political.

These tensions are further seen in Ajay's account, highlighted by the changing position of the drug, heroin, from 'golden brown' to a 'brown bitch'. Like in Lucy's account, Ajay starts off by conceptualising heroin in terms of pleasure, but it quickly becomes about something more (or less). I asked: 'And then how does that make your body feel?'. Referring to the body map he had just drawn, Ajay replied: 'Right…shall I do another one [body map]?' He explains that his first picture (on the right-hand side of Figure 2.1) is about before using drugs: 'so this is before: "waiting for your dealer", yeah'. And his new one depicts 'after, this would be, "after", "under the influence"'. He then started writing some song lyrics (see the left-hand side of Figure 2.1), and said: 'It's true – have you heard it – golden brown, texture like sun, lays me down with my mind she runs, throughout the night, no need to fight, never a frown with golden brown'. With this, he demonstrated a relaxed look, singing the song with his eyes half shut, with a slight swaying of his head and upper body. This provoked some laughter between us, and after I confirmed

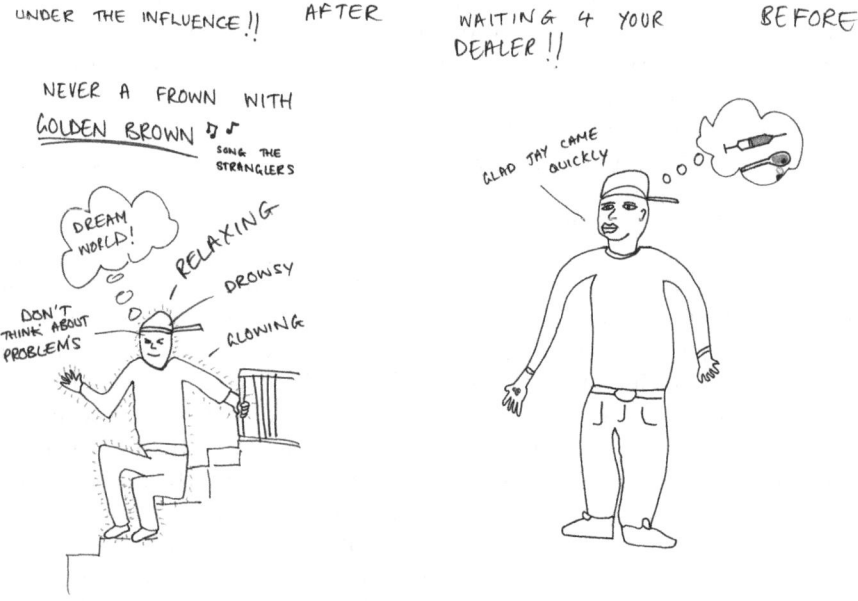

Figure 2.1 Ajay's body map.

that I knew the song, he continued to sing it to me, that is, before, much like with Lucy's description, another thought made itself known:

> dud dud dud dud dud dud, dud dud dud dud dud dud (singing and swaying to the keyboard vamps in 3/4 bar). *Right*, or, I call her my brown (stops himself to explain), obviously it's a love/hate relationship with drug use... I call her a (pause) brown bitch, to be honest, because obviously she causes you so much pain but you still go running back to her, it's like a woman that makes you feel good when you're around her, she makes you feel good, but if you're without her, you're love sick, you're sick as a dog, you can't function without her, you're cold, you're sneezing, yeah, but when she's around you, you feel happy and when she's, like, when you're under the influence and you're wrapped around her, all you think about is her and you're happy to be in contact with her but when she leaves you, you're love sick and you'll do anything, you'll do anything to get the feeling back, but yeah, heroin is a woman that treats me bad, *but I still love her* (emphasis put on this). Do you understand? (Ajay)

Ajay's exposition vividly highlights some of the complexities caught up in participants' feelings towards their drug use. He started off describing the feeling of heroin through the song lyrics and rhythms of 'golden brown', and affectively re-enacts the pleasures of being 'under the influence'. But then, like Lucy, he suddenly stops, as if again being cut off, and says 'right'. This again invokes the notion that thoughts are not our own – the pleasurable memories escape him (to reuse Matt's statement, he has 'forgotten how it was to enjoy [his] use'), and he starts to remember the bad side, or in Lucy's terms, 'the crap'. For Ajay, this is namely the role of dependency (connected to a concept of addiction as antithetical to pleasure), which he personifies as 'girlfriend-like', perhaps to communicate a non-human agency that is otherwise hard to explain (a device also used by other participants). Drawing on this agency, he proceeded to poetically tell me about his conflict with the substance he loves, but causes him so much pain. In feminising the drug, he also affirms that this experience is not divorced from sociopolitical structures.

The idea that pleasure can live outside the 'crap' (as freely chosen) makes little sense; instead it moves through networks, always in 'passing' (Deleuze and Guattari, 1994: 109; Gomart and Hennion, 1999). In the interviews, participants would sometimes say there was no pleasure in their drug use, it was purely 'addiction', and then they realised there was also pleasure, or like in Ajay's and Lucy's account, would start off thinking about their drug use as simply pleasure-orientated and then talk about addiction. Earlier in the interview Ajay said: 'I use drugs because I enjoy using drugs, that's the only reason I do use drugs'. This was later reinforced with: 'I use because I want to use, not because I'm a street junkie, I use because I enjoy using'. But then, he realised there was also 'so much pain'. Like in Matt's initial response (above) and my observations of the drug service, this lack of pleasure is more than a performance or role. Thinking *about* pleasure is hard because the bodies that condition it are often the same bodies that have also been affected by concepts of addiction, and it is concepts of addiction, plugged into the scientific apparatuses seen above, that are likely to make themselves known more forcefully and powerfully.

Participants would talk about how their drug use started off as pleasurable and then they got 'hooked'. Dimitri says, 'I really enjoyed it and it's all good, the enjoyment's good until like you're hooked. And then when you're hooked, it's a different story'. However, pleasure would then emerge somewhere else in the interview. It was hard to keep the positive and negative affects apart. Matias, for example, was talking about his 'dependency' when the 'taste' and 'feeling' entered:

> It's not just the dependency, you want to, I don't know, when you inject, I don't know, you feel the taste in your throat and then the feeling that comes down on you, I don't know, it's quite enjoyable. It's I suppose like smoking opium, I've never done it, but I imagine it's the same anyway, and as I said you keep on trying to get that which you felt years ago, and you don't anymore because it's so downer (referring to the sleeping tablets which he feels are now extensively mixed in with the heroin).

These tensions were conceptualised by Lucy as 'mixed feelings', but others described similar feelings as a 'love/hate relationship' (Ajay), 'sweet and sour' (Reggie) and 'good things and bad things' (Simon). Simon says: 'how bad it was but also how nice it was at the same time' This resonates with the 'pharmakon' as both poison and remedy (Fraser and Moore, 2011; Fraser and valentine, 2008; Keane, 2002; Rinella, 2010). But not only do the positions of 'poison' and 'remedy' struggle, but so too do the subject and object positions. Ajay's account questions any predefined object/subject or structure/agency positions – the subject and object seem to come into being through the event. Heroin moves from an object (golden *brown*) to a subject (brown *bitch*). This chimes with Colebrook's analysis of Deleuze's 'becoming' as 'desire': 'The "who" or "what" that desires (the distinction between inside and outside) is produced in and through the production of relations' (Colebrook, 2002: 117).

To conclude this chapter, I hope to have shown how through participants' conceptualisation practices, pleasure is produced as antithetical to addiction, but true to its construction, it is also collapsed. Furthermore, as the antithetical dynamic of pleasure/addiction started to show itself up in this way as a modern paradox, I was able to understand some of the complexities of what the participants were telling me in a way that did not rely on such binaries. Consequently, by thinking with Deleuze and Guattari's body that thinks and concepts that act, and Latour's Modern Constitution, I have been able to get closer to the tensions that underpin drugged pleasures in a material yet political way (caught up in human-non-human networks) as only ever partial. In participants' partial affinities with drugs, drugs and their networks are not connected with (thought about) in an abstract way but are part of the conditions of thought that make them knowable. By taking these tensions seriously, I hope to encourage new ways of conceptualising drugged pleasures beyond restrictive divides like objective/subjective, recreational/dependent, mental/physical, so pleasure can play a bigger role in drug service provision. Workers who are currently actively turning away from or trying to manage pleasure should turn towards it and pay attention to it, including asking questions about pleasure and being open to people's responses (Gonçalves et al., 2016). It is through such curiosity that workers will be able to help bring about more generative, 'healthier' forms of pleasure. Tensions are not something to be feared, as a lack of certainty, but followed as we seek to acknowledge and potentialise different and more productive experiences. Continuing to 'stay with the trouble', as Haraway (2013; 2016) would have us do, I will next look at some other tensions in practising bodies in the injecting event.

Notes

1 Pleasure remains neglected in studies of addictive drug use, with some notable exceptions, including Dwyer (2008), Harris and Rhodes (2012), Pienaar et al. (2015).
2 Mainstream calls to include a discussion of pleasure in drug research, policy and treatment frequently exclude drugs such as heroin and crack cocaine. See, for example, Global Drug Survey's Pleasure Index, and Nutt's (2012) commentary.
3 Ambivalence is a term used in drug services to describe a service user's uncertainty about whether they want to give up drugs.
4 For example, during my time at the service, the stairwell was painted from dark green to a paler tone, and I spent several hours helping a worker to make one of the rooms adjacent to the main building feel more 'therapeutic' for counselling sessions, including re-arranging furniture and putting up attractive posters.

Chapter 3

Practicing bodies

'On the tilt': the injecting event and the fragility of pleasure amongst other affects

Pleasure is a fragile accomplishment.

Kane Race, 2008: 420

I suppose it's like having the worst hunger or anything and, or, you haven't had a drink for days and then you get water, and it's almost as if it [the glass] could drop over any minute, so you're really thirsty, so it's on the tilt, but if you get it then your replenished, but if you miss it then it's on the floor. So, it's the same if you miss a hit.

Lucy, 42 years old, injects heroin

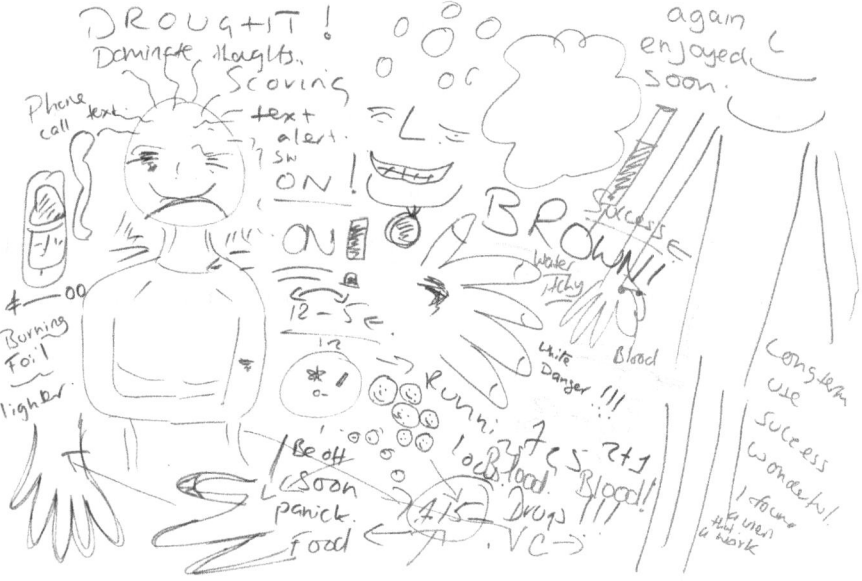

Figure 3.1 Lucy's body map.

Where Chapter 2 looked at how pleasure was conceptualised as always in tension, this chapter attends to these tensions in the injecting event itself. I will look at the relational makeup of the injecting event in which pleasure, amongst other slippery affects, is enacted through a fragile assemblage of bodies (human and non-human). The fragility of this assemblage is encapsulated in Lucy's metaphor of the tilting water glass, where the injecting event is seen as beyond her control ('could drop over at any minute'), contingent on the precise coming together of bodies, things and forces. Lucy's body map (Figure 3.1) explores these arrays. Where I asked her to map her body, a much more relational understanding of the embodied injecting event gets depicted. Lucy writes the words 'long term use success, wonderful', which sums up a long discussion, aided through the drawing, on the fragility of the injecting event (compounded by many years of injecting), and the 'wonderful' feelings when it is successful. From the picture, it is clear that this 'success' is made up of several tentative actors and connections. The mobile phone, with 'text alerts' from her dealer stating when he is 'on' and 'running low', produces and interacts with her 'dominant thoughts'. Her hands 'remind' her of injecting and provide her only accessible veins for injecting. A clock/watch is central to knowing the time when the dealer is 'on' (12–5pm), and 'triggers' her desire to use. Also present is the money (£15), substance itself ('brown'), syringe and 'cooker'. The dealer and other people at the dealer's location are drawn as the faces in the picture. These components of the mapped body could be read as symbolic for a line of events leading up to the injection, but I think this would be too neat. Rather, again, 'staying with the trouble' (the tensions), I try to stay with and explore the sense of muddle, mess and ambiguity in the injecting event, that is, things seem to suddenly come together, but can just as easily shift and fall apart ('drop'), which points towards its fragility: 'there's this 50/50 if it's going to work, 50 heaven, 50 hell' (Lucy). 'Success' is based on a finely attuned balancing act of various actants, so that to assume Lucy and other participants an active role in relation to the passivity of their tools (mastery over their tools/environment) would be to underplay their coproduction.

Using Lucy's drawing (Figure 3.1) and accompanying narrative as my starting point, to be fleshed out with other participants' accounts, this chapter explores pleasure (rather than subjective or objective, freely chosen or of the mechanical body) as a relational achievement. The first section underpins this conceptual shift in relation to Latour's (1999a) and Gomart and Hennion's (1999) 'sociology of attachments', which is positioned in contrast to Howard Becker's understanding of drugs' pleasures as a *social accomplishment*. The second section maps these attachments through the sociomaterial pleasure assemblage. The third section pays particular attention to the *preparatory work* involved in securing these attachments 'successfully'. The third and fourth sections explore *what happens* when this success is achieved, but also what happens when the connections become too fragile and the metaphorical glass drops. Pleasure in this sense is permanently 'on the tilt', and 'keeping the glass upright' has become a task of life for many of the participants. The final section will zero in on 'the speedball' as a particularly fragile attachment, exemplifying pleasure as a relational achievement.

Keeping the glass upright: a relational achievement

In his groundbreaking essay, 'Becoming a Marihuana User', American sociologist Howard Becker proposed that smoking marijuana was not a simple pharmacokinetic process, but rather learnt as a social accomplishment, based on practice and peer negotiation. By linking marihuana use to social practice, these findings refuted a longstanding position that such use and, by extension, other kinds of drug use were due to behavioural disposition or pathology and thus could start to be imagined as a sociological issue rather than a biological or criminal one. He accounted for how people become regular users of cannabis by learning to perceive it as pleasurable. Pleasure in this sense is far from a natural or objective phenomenon – the substance interacting with the brain/body – but is rather learnt in a process of assigning meaning to the smoking experience: 'it is only when he [sic] can do this that he is high' (Becker, 1953: 238).

For Becker, 'getting high' is reliant on a cognitive reconceptualisation of experience, where the subject is centre stage. The drug user is put in control of their drug use, defining whether it is pleasurable or not, and by implication whether they will rationally continue. Becker describes a three-step process in which this learning takes place:

> An individual will be able to use marihuana for pleasure only when he (1) learns to smoke it in a way that will produce real effects; (2) learns to recognize the effects and connect them with drug use; and (3) learns to enjoy the sensations he perceives.
>
> (1953: 235)

This process of learning to use marijuana for pleasure is what Kane Race refers to in Becker's thesis as a 'fragile accomplishment' (2008: 420). However, in my study, the fragility seemed to be coming from elsewhere. This was less about an individual accomplishment (albeit acquired through social interaction) and more about a relationally sociomaterial achievement.[1] In this shift, I take up Race's (2008) pre-emption, and perhaps even invitation, for a 'more contemporary reading' of pleasure, in following Latour's (1999a) and Gomart and Hennion's (1999) 'sociology of attachment', to rethink these practices in a more relational way. Pleasure seemed to be reliant on a delicate coming together of various bodies, human and not, where the slightest slip could lead to the whole assemblage collapsing (the glass being dropped), and hence, Lucy's feeling that it was always 'on the tilt'.

To push the analogy of the tilting water glass further, it seemed that many 'actants' (human and non-human actors) were involved in keeping it upright: keeping the injecting assemblage together in a way that could enact pleasure. This understanding has been helped by an article written by Latour (1999a) on smoking. In the article, Latour discusses a comic strip. A man is smoking and his daughter asks 'what are you doing', he replies 'I'm smoking', at which she says 'I thought the cigarette was smoking you'. The father is thrown into panic and chops his cigarettes up. Latour argues that the binaries of passive/active have been turned on their head – is it the subject who is in control of the object (cigarette) or the cigarette (object) who is in control of the subject? But, instead, Latour suggests neither:

> There is nothing in this resembling a determining action, neither for it nor for me. I do not control it any more than it controls me. I am *attached* to it, and if I cannot hope for any kind of emancipation from it, then perhaps other attachments will come to substitute for this one, on condition that I don't panic and that you do not, as a good critical sociology of the left would, impose upon me an ideal of detachment from which I would surely perish. [...] We can substitute one attachment for another, but we cannot move from a state of attachment to that of unattachment. This is what a father should tell his daughter. To understand the activity of subjects, their emotions, *their passions,* we must turn our attention to *that which attaches and activates them* – an obvious proposition, but one normally overlooked.
>
> (1999a: 27, my emphasis)

In this entertaining way, Latour is suggesting that we move away from positions of active/passive and structure/agency, and instead turn to what attaches us. That same year, inspired by Latour and other's actor-network theory, Emilie Gomart and Antoine Hennion (1999) draw our sociological attention to drug users' attachments and their strategies to be actively 'seized by objects' in their 'passing' between agency and passivity. Again, this is not a case of mastery (the drug's or the user's), but rather an emergence of an 'impassioned' event – 'making oneself available' (disposed) to 'the socio-technical "dispositifs" of passion' (1999: 221).

I now turn to this 'dispositif of passion' or the pleasure assemblage, before developing this argument further in the following section regarding how participants, in their connection to others, make themselves available to it – to become 'impassioned'.

The pleasure assemblage

Pleasure as a relational achievement involved an assemblage of injecting bodies that I look at here in terms of substances (methadone, buprenorphine, Valium and alcohol), 'paraphernalia', people and space-time.

For some participants, methadone, a commonly prescribed opiate substitute for heroin dependency, formed a key part of the pleasure assemblage, but in very different ways. This is interesting because methadone is purposely designed to inhibit pleasure; to be taken to stave off withdrawals only and even re-discipline drug users through its administration routines into mainstream society (Bourgois, 2000). However, for Paula, like others, methadone could explicitly bring about a 'better hit [high from injecting heroin]':

> But then you do the methadone and take the stuff [heroin] as well, get a better hit (*laughs*). I'm sorry but that's what you did, you got a better hit.

Interestingly, she nervously laughs and apologises for linking methadone to pleasure, a connection that is not supposed to be made (Bourgois, 2000).

But, where for Paula, methadone brought about a 'better hit', for other participants, it constrained pleasure, and the 'success' of the injecting assemblage became more reliant on an absence of methadone. For example, Jim would 'swipe a load of methadone away', enduring the uncomfortable withdrawal symptoms ('clucking'), in order to induce a 'real big hit':

> When your system is soaked with methadone, a bit of heroin, you don't even feel it, and the same with diamorphine [pharmaceutical heroin]. If I come out and have a hit, it covers the heroin, and even if they put my methadone up so high, I wouldn't feel the diamorphine. If I didn't have any methadone in my system and I had this hit, I'd feel it… So what I'd try and do is swipe a load of methadone away, wait until I'm clucking, and then buy a load of it [street heroin], and then I'd get a *real big hit off it.*

Similar attachments were reported in relation to buprenorphine, which was the second-most common opiate substitute used in treatment at both drug services and in the UK more generally (methadone being the first). But as a partial antagonist-agonist to the opioid receptors, as opposed to methadone which is a full agnostic, these findings are perhaps even more interesting because buprenorphine could send the recipient into immediate withdrawals if combined with heroin. As such, buprenorphine was only recommended for those service users deemed to be serious about giving up their heroin consumption. However, conversely, Dimitri explains a system of mediation practices in which he had worked out the optimum dose and time to take his buprenorphine to maximise the feeling from his heroin use.

> So this is what I was doing last summer, I was taking my 8 ml [of buprenorphine] in the morning and then 12 o'clock in the afternoon, when a dealer come on, I'd get a bag of gear [heroin], and then I'd be in the park or wherever all day and then when I go home, I went until 9 o'clock at night, and then I'll do the bag of gear and then I'd really feel it.

Interestingly, this meant that, against the common belief amongst service providers that buprenorphine is better at reducing 'on top' heroin use, due to its 'blocking' (partial antagonist) formula, Dimitri actually found himself using more heroin than he did when he was on methadone.

> When I was on the methadone, I was on 60ml, and anything over 50ml, you don't really feel the heroin, so therefore, I could leave it alone for months, and not do it, but now that I'm on the Subutex (brand name for buprenorphine), I know that if I don't take Subutex, I'm gonna feel the gear, and so I've been using more since.

For other participants, the stakes of this negotiation were felt to be too high. If the balance was not negotiated with extreme care, the fragile mix of heroin and buprenorphine could precipitate withdrawals, which, for Tom, made it an impossible alternative to methadone:

> You couldn't do that, you couldn't use [heroin] on top. Years ago, I had terrible troubles with Subutex. I sort of went to get clean, got down to about 10 mil of methadone and then went onto buprenorphine cos it's got the blocker [partial antagonist] in it supposedly. But then, so I ended up taking buprenorphine just for the blocker, but I found the transition horrible, and then I found out that the blocker only works for about 4 hours so then *when I found myself* using [heroin] on top, I found it *fucking murder*. Switching to buprenorphine, I found it really hard. It just ended up being a waste of a script. I think methadone is much easier.

Here, there is a sense that methadone can better cope with the injecting assemblage, that is, the sudden coming together of things, in which Tom 'found [himself] using on top'. This is an interesting choice of words, which stresses the workings of an event rather than an individual agent. Tom preferred methadone as it allowed for those assemblic moments when he *found* himself using. Buprenorphine, on the other hand, did not have such contingency. This speaks to Hennion's idea of making oneself open to being moved, without controlling it: 'What should happen is not planned or intentional: we must allow ourselves to be carried away, moved, so that something can take place' (2001:12).

Using similar language, Jim talks about being literally moved, indeed, almost transplanted, by Valium (brand name for the sedative, diazepam). He refers to Valium as the 'charge sheet' because after taking several tablets, he says, people often find themselves in a police cell, facing a criminal charge, with no recollection of how they got there.

> Valium, really, when I first started taking it, when I got into it as a teenager, it was brilliant, I could go out shoplifting and I would, it was literally like I was invisible, and the thing is, it did work. I was literally caning it, getting a few hundred quid a day, I was just so, *it just inspired*

me to do everything, and I was just doing everything, everything, and I was just doing everything that I wanted to do. It's not even like I was getting caught, people call them the 'charge sheets', Valium, because they take a load of Valium and wake up in the station, they don't really know exactly what got them there, that's generally what happens. And like I said your confidence is amazing. Girls that I wouldn't think of approaching, I could chat them up and I would get off with them. It would be different if you tried but then didn't, but you do.

It is with drug use in mind that Gomart and Hennion (1999) argue that passivity is not always a negative asset, an absence of capacity, but rather can actually produce creativity: '"constraints" become the generous aspects of things which, if prepared for, create existence and initiate transformation' (1999: 221). For Jim, Valium enabled or 'inspired' him 'to do everything', which could bring about pleasure (e.g. 'getting off' with a girl), but could also tip over into a criminal charge. He stresses that Valium did not just make him feel like he could do things, but he actually could do these things – 'it would be different if you tried but then didn't, but you do'. The induced passivity is therefore anything but inactive. Gomart (2002a; 2004), in her lone work, extends this argument in relation to methadone: 'human agency is tentatively and temporarily re-defined as the capacity not to act alone, but [...] to act because one was generously constrained' (2002a: 546). In Jim's case, it was his passivity to being moved by Valium that meant he could actually do want he wanted. For Mike (below), Valium was particularly powerful in producing passivity ('total obliteration') which could bring him pleasure ('I've always liked the way they make me feel') or at least an absence of pain ('killed my pain'), but also could encourage him to use other drugs or commit criminal offenses. This was both a source of pleasure and concern of which he now 'tend[s] to stay away from'.

I will now quote quite extensively from our conversation as it captures the ambiguity of the active-passive process.

FD: So, have benzos [benzodiazepines], Valium and that, been a big part of your drug use?

MIKE: Yeah it has, because I've always liked them. I've always liked the way they make me feel, and the effect that they give.

FD: Can you say more?

MIKE: Well they just, it's just total obliteration. What I got from heroin, the way it killed my pain and it sort of drained away all my worries and you know, all my problems and that, although temporarily. The benzos is something else, it just stops your brain functioning altogether, *you've got like 1 per cent brain function, your just walking around unconscious,* you don't feel nothing, you don't even feel pain, the amount of injuries I've got on those things, I've smashed my elbows, my knees, I've like fallen over, smashed my face on the floor, all sorts. You don't feel no pain, you're just walking around like... it's dangerous; that's why I tend to stay away from them now.

FD: Would you walk around rather than just stay in?

MIKE: Well you'd think you'd stay in because you're all sleepy, like drowsy and that, you'd think you'd just stay in and like sit in front of the TV or whatever, and sometimes I'll do that. If I'm on a benzo binge, I'll like, sometimes I'll get some cannabis and I'll just be sitting there, I'll roll a joint, smoke some of it, put it down in the ashtray, maybe nod off for two hours, and then I'll wake up and they've worn off me a little bit, but I've got a whole bottle of tablets there so I'll eat a few more, light a joint up and go back to sleep again. But other times they can make you, like alcohol, they remove your inhibitions and they make you crave for other things, so sometimes you think oh I could really do with a hit right now, that would be really great. Or you, they can also drive you to go out and commit criminal offenses, all sorts...

FD: But I bet you're not the best criminal when you're...?

MIKE: Nah, you think you are, it's like you're walking around and you think you're invisible, but you're not, you're standing out like a sore thumb [laughing]. Well I say it's funny but it's not. It always ends badly. It's amazing like the thing you get, you're creeping around like no one can see ya, it's pretty crazy.

Valium brought about an active-passivity (epitomised in the paradoxical notion of 'walking around unconscious') that allowed both Mike and Jim to do things they would not have otherwise thought of doing (e.g. 'approaching girls').

It is this same quality that made Valium, for some, a key part of the injecting assemblage – to become 'impassioned'. For example, Simon notes how it brought about his injecting:

> The other thing is sometimes I might, which is kind of silly, but I'm trying to watch out for it, I mean I do watch out for it, I don't do it... I'm not silly, but sometimes I'll take a Valium as well and that might sometimes lead to me having a hit.

Simon goes on to explain how Valium enables the body to open up, to actively receive pleasure: 'your body starts to go in on itself, so the Valium [...] makes you relaxed'. Where, for Simon, like Mike, Valium was part of the assemblage which could move him towards a 'hit', for others it took on an even more pivotal role in enacting pleasure, in stabilising the metaphorical glass and enhancing the capabilities of other substances. For example, Valium could take the 'edginess' off the crack cocaine or speedball: 'it goes well with the white [crack], it sort of balances it, because it relaxes you, so you don't get that kind of edgy' (Silvie). And, it could enhance the desired 'gouchiness' of the heroin: 'what it does, it also makes like the heroin stronger, it sort of, it interacts, it sort of brings the heroin on more... and so like you do feel more like gouchy off it' (Dimitri).

Alcohol acts in a similar way. This resonates with Demant's (2009) important article on 'when alcohol acts' at teenage parties. Rather than being led by users' perceptions of alcohol, Demant considers the role of alcohol itself in producing a 'pleasure-filled body' (Demant, 2009: 35). For many participants here, alcohol had become an essential part of keeping the injecting assemblage together ('keeping the glass upright') in a way that could enact pleasure. For Mason, he had to drink a lot of beer before he was able to enjoy the heroin and fall asleep:

> I will lie down eventually, but I drink a lot of beer first. When I'm able to, see I can't sleep, even without drugs, I can't sleep. But that is why this gives me the ability to actually lie down and sleep. So that is the end result that I want when I do it [heroin].

Alcohol helps the pleasure assemblage *work* by maximising the effects of the heroin and minimising the stress of finding a 'next fix' ('chasing my tail'):

> Like I said, the only thing I do is alcohol cos it *makes the gear work*, and more for economics than anything else, because I don't want to keep on chasing my tail. If I'm going to do it, there's no point stressing myself out about where I'm going to get my next fix, there's too many people that do that, and that's why I don't hang around with people, because I like to be able to sit down, read a book, and concentrate my mind on other things rather than just running around chasing my tail and trying to make money, d'you know what I mean.

With this, Mason hints at the issue of trying to separate these actants out, as the role of alcohol is at once part of something much bigger. Reaching the desired end point is not only produced by heroin and alcohol, but by being alone and 'able to sit down, [and] read a book'. Alcohol is key to producing affects other than addiction. He uses it precisely in order to endure a passivity conducive to pleasure rather than addiction or what he calls 'chasing his tail'.

What is undoubtedly an obvious part of the assemblage, but perhaps one that often gets overlooked, is the injecting equipment or paraphernalia, including the needle-syringe, water, citric or vitamin C, filter, cooker, lighter, etc. Such are crucial to the injecting event and its 'successful' enactment of pleasure. But where these are more commonly, especially in public health literature, discussed as facilitating human action, I try to look at them as actors in their own right.

Starting with the syringe, participants often spoke of 'the needle fixation'. However, on further enquiry, the phrase seemed more figurative, plugging-in to a long and fiercely debated discourse within public health and promulgated in treatment services (Fraser et al., 2004; Vitellone, 2003b; 2017). Participants' use of the term appears to denote a desire to articulate a close relationship with the needle rather than a pathological one. For Lucy, it seems to be a way of expressing how the needle is a common part of her life, not as a 'fixation', but as a key actant in the injecting event and in experiencing 'the hit' (discussed further below). Dimitri even says: 'well I'm not actually fixated'. The needle is central to the intensity of the injecting experience, beyond its capacity to deliver the heroin quicker. For example, Meg says: 'Once you've started injecting, *the whole thing* of it is really, the whole needle thing, it just doesn't seem to work when you smoke it, you need to inject it once you've started'.

Once these bodies (needle, paraphernalia, 'genetic body') have come together (described as a 'ritual'), there is a sense of no going back, the needle has become central to the intracorporeality (this is discussed in terms of habit in Chapter 5). Drawing on Vitellone's (2003a; 2003b; 2010; 2015; 2017) repeated calls to take the syringe seriously, I suggest here that the needle[2] is a body in the same way as the human body. Where sociality has been stressed in some sociological studies of drug-using communities (the 'drug set' in Zinberg's [1984] classic study), here the needle is just as important. Meg goes on to explain that 'once you're used to that' connection, that is, your addiction:

> It's like, how to put it, it just doesn't feel the same smoking it, it's much stronger, you get an instant hit when you inject it – when you smoke it, it's more gradual – so it's an instant hit, so once you're used to that, *that's your addiction*, do you know what I mean, that's what you're looking for. So when you're smoking, *it's not hitting the spot*, it's not, you're not feeling it, it doesn't do it.

And this is why, for Meg, an opiate substitute, taken orally, did not work:

> That's why I carried on doing it even though I had methadone so I wasn't actually sick but there's still something missing, you still feel like, because it's a different drug, it's not the same thing, so you still want a hit, you want the instant element.

The bodies of the needle, drug and biological (venous, nervous, neurological) system come together to create a 'different drug' – it is at this point of intra-action that the site of addiction lies, rather than with the disconnected substance (e.g. heroin). (This point is further elaborated and exemplified in participants' accounts of the 'speedball' below).

For some participants, there was pleasure found in the pain of piercing the skin, but also concerns around this pleasure, for example, Silvie cautiously states:

> It's kind of like, doing something to yourself, even if you know ... I don't know, it's strange... because the pleasure is coming, but in a way you have to kind of hurt yourself a little bit, even if it doesn't hurt that much, it's kind of, not self-harming, but you know what I'm trying to say.

This is similar to the way that Lucy problematises the role of the 'itchy' ('uncomfortable'), but yet pleasurable (knowing the hit has been successful) position of the citric acid that is used for dissolving the heroin.

> Citric gives an itchy sensation but you know when you get this itchy, it's weird, it's actually uncomfortable, but you know that you've had a successful hit. Even if you go, oh itchy, I need to go and wash my hand, it's like intense pins and needles, you know that the citric has gone in, it's gone in, it's worked, so you know that soon after you're starting to do that (she drops her head, enacting 'nodding off'). Even though you're annoyed, it's a horrible itchy feeling, because it's the citric going into your veins, with vitamin c it's less itchy, but what I've noticed with the itchy feeling is the success. It always means it's pulled well, it hasn't hurt and it's worked, so success. So 'itchy, success' (writes it on her body map) and then I'd go to water cos I'd wash my hands because they feel itchy but then success, so I'm smiling.

The citric acid plays a pivotal role in letting Lucy know that the injection has worked, and the itchy feeling was constitutive of this realisation and making it real, rather than being merely facilitative. It simultaneously registers and materialises the 'success'.

Adding to what has so far been described as a largely non-human assemblage, other human bodies, or the lack of, also played an important role in the injecting event and whether pleasure was reached or not. For some, it was only in being around other injectors that they would inject: 'But even now I can stop doing that and smoke it, if I'm not around other injectors, I will do that' (Gwen). The role of peers was particularly important when it came to starting injecting. Most participants recalled a situation in which they were initiated into injecting by intrigue or encouragement from other injectors, or in a situation in which they were experiencing withdrawals and only around people who had injectable opiates. In terms of enacting pleasure, human company was also seen to be able to direct the drug-using experience towards something more pleasurable.

In Anita's case, this was away from 'cleaning' and 'chasing' to something more comforting:

> I'm always with that one girlfriend round me you know. I like to have company, I really do, like, on my own it's like I go on a cleaning buzz or a mad run or a, d'you know what I mean, I just want more and more, I start chasing it and everything but if I have someone, I like to talk to someone, *I like that whole situation.*

I interviewed (separately) at least one romantic couple, Crystal and Mike, and two sets of friends who injected together, Jim and Carlos, and Gwen and Sandra. Their relationships were important for the 'successful' coming-together of the event in itself, for example, in getting the money together, scoring the drugs, 'cooking up', helping each other to inject, etc., but also in enacting pleasure and, in both cases, with this, came safety. Jim says:

> I think most of the time, now, I do like a bit of company cos when I'm on my own I can get very down, very depressed, and that's mainly, if I've got a lot of gear, I start like put three bits of white, two browns or you know, doing a lot, lot more, and I wouldn't think of the consequences. Whereas when you're with a mate, you don't do so much, we might split it.

Interestingly, Jim had recently started a diamorphine programme,[3] which meant his consumption of heroin had started to reduce, and with this, Carlos had also started to reduce his. This stresses the relationality of addiction and challenges dominant models of addiction as an individual disease. Carlos says:

> Actually, I start cutting down a little since he started the diamorphine, because before we were together 24 hours and we would just say bye at 2 or 3 o'clock in the morning when he would go up to his bed, sorry, I would go up to my room, but then next day, we wake up, have breakfast and then we go out and make money or whatever so we'd be out. But now, he's taking his diamorphine, we only meet once in a while so I'm cutting down a good. Before, by now, I would have had 4–5 hits, so today I've had two, I've still had two, but not bad.

Emphasising this shift further, Carlos says:

> For example, before, we're talking about a month ago, with this money now (reimbursement for the interview), what I would do, I would try to go out straight away, make another £10, with this money for buying another 1:1 [1 bag of heroin: 1 bag of crack], with this money I would think

about another hit, but, now, what I'm going to do, is with this money, I'm going to buy a Freeview (to watch television).

I ask again about what brought this change about, and Carlos replies:

One, I take my medication. Two, I took two hits today. And three I'm alone, it's good to have that feeling, it's a good feeling, but when you have that person that is one, pulling money as well and two, enjoys the same buzz.

Carlos's injecting was evidently entwined with Jim's – the shared work going in, such as earning the money and scoring – but also the shared results:

FD: You would enjoy the buzz together?
CARLOS: Yeah, yeah
FD: So you could chat?
CARLOS: Exactly. I'm a very chatty, chatty boy when I take.
FD: Jim is chatty as well? So both of you…
CARLOS: It's like 'let me speak, let me speak' (he imitates the speed). It's quite great. It's nice.

Other participants reflected on a shift in the intracorporeal relationships involved in injecting, which during the preparatory stage were more shared with the materials ('doing their own thing'), and then the 'buzzing' was shared with the group. Reggie says that, after scoring

we'll come back and just start cooking up and then everyone's got their own needles and that so like basically what you do is, you get a spoon and that yeah and you put it in, you get your citric acid, yeah, then you put a little bit of water, then you boil it and then you get err either a cigarette butt and pull it out of a filter and put it, let in soak it up and then stick your needle in it and then draw it up. So everyone's like there doing their own thing, *but then we're all like buzzing together* sort of thing.

For some participants, having people or friends around was more than company, but a necessity at a pragmatic level. It was common for partners or friends to help with their injecting, and they often spoke highly of their technique and skill. In following a sociology of attachment, the participants' partners/friends can be seen as helping to constitute the injecting event and their 'becoming-together' as an 'injecting drug user', even if the injection was performed by somebody else.

In the act of tasting, in the gestures that allow it, in the know-how that accompanies it, in the supports sought (*in other people*, or in guides and reviews), in the tiny ongoing adjustments that lay it out and favour its felicity and reproducibility – it is on the basis of all these responses that objects return to those who take an interest in them.

(Hennion, 2007: 101, my emphasis)

It is these very intimacies that invigorate Vitellone's (2015; 2017) recent work on the *Social Science of the Syringe* and the relationships the syringe can produce (see also Hart, 2018; Duff, 2018, for commentaries). This is perhaps why so many participants said that if their drug use was to end, their relationships with their partners would come under threat or undo completely, and vice versa, if their relationship ended. For example, Meg says: 'I don't even know what's going to happen once we're finally off everything, because I think it's probably just drugs holding everything together'. Similarly, for Gwen, she recalled how, when her friend who she relied on to inject her went into prison, she went back to smoking heroin.

Conversely, for other participants, human company disrupted 'the so-called buzz'. Therefore, rather than desiring or needing company, being alone became a constitutive feature of enacting pleasure. Grigor says:

So, me, I started not associating with people because I was so fed up because the so-called buzz or euphoria that you're having is you can't enjoy because some other people. They'll be an argument or something so I started going by myself, really staying away from people.

A similar avoidance of volatility was expressed in terms of where and when participants used. The 'crack house' was one particular configuration of space and time that could often erupt. For Reggie (see Figure 3.2), this meant he could not relax, which substantially reduced his 'gouching' period: 'If I'm with people in a crack house, I don't really know them and that, then I can't relax in there'. The crack house actively effects the gouching time. This ties in with more recent theorisations of drug contexts in which space and time are seen as co-constitutive (e.g. Bøhling, 2014; Duff, 2007; 2012; Farrugia, 2015; Fraser, 2006; Race, 2014). Context is redefined as not something the drug user is within, but something that gets made, to different effects (harmful, pleasurable, etc.), in the using event.

In Reggie's account of the crack house, he could not gain the active-passivity required to become truly impassioned. This is why participants often cited being at 'home' as one of the key space-times for pleasure to exist. When I asked Lucy about where she tends to use, she emphatically says: 'definitely at home, it's like a ritual at home'. But for Lucy, like many women, this space was also vulnerable to getting encroached on by drug dealers, who threatened her capacity to enjoy the hit. But, worse still, it also produced particularly exploitative arrangements of space-time: 'they're chopping up and doing up their bags and they'll only give you like two

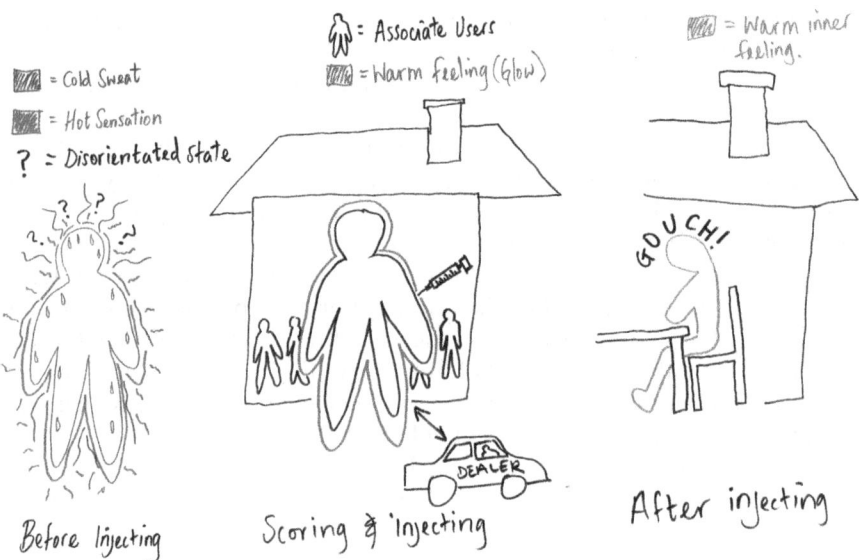

Figure 3.2 Reggie's body map. He has to move from the 'crack house' (second scene) to somewhere else (third scene) in order to enjoy the 'gouch'. The 'gouch' is notably only when he is sitting down, which the chair affords.

£7.50 bits [crack/heroin] for doing it, so £15 for misusing your flat' (Gwen). In employing Barad's (2007) notion of subjectivity as intra-relational, particular subject positions vulnerable to exploitation were being produced. Lucy recounts a situation in which she was forced to endanger herself in order to buy the Valium that her doctor refused to prescribe. In this sense, like with Suzanne Fraser's (2006) cautionary tale of drug service's involvement in the production of 'dependent' methadone clients, the medical team that ignored Lucy's call for help are not immune from this subject production-site. (This is a point that I return to in Chapter 5.)

To recapitulate, I have highlighted how pleasure as a relational achievement is brought into being through a 'repertoire' of bodies, human and not. Rather than seeing objects as facilitative of human agency/activity in seeking pleasure and other drug effects, I have tried to address them as part of this assemblage in their own right. But, running throughout this section has been a sense of the fragility of these object-subject connections – 'on the tilt' – and hence I turn now to the techno-corporeal techniques involved in preparing and directing bodies towards these attachments.

Fragile connections: directing bodies towards pleasure

> Since the connection is not permanent, nor strong, but rather partial and fragile it has therefore to be nurtured and cultivated with care.
>
> Morgan Meyer, 2008: 48

> Once it is singled out as a topic of study, even undergoing appears to have little to do with being passive. It is hard work. Ask amateurs – of music, of drugs, of wine – and follow what they do in practice. They do a lot: their pleasure depends on preparations.
>
> Annemarie Mol, 2010: 256

The affects felt by injecting drugs are not something that are simply done by the drugs but something that are contingent on the coming together of many bodies and forces. But these attachments are fragile, and work has to be done to keep them together – to keep the glass upright. Although I touched on this in the previous section, I want to now elaborate further on the precise nature of some of this work being done to keep these fragile connections together. Rather than looking at the discursive practices of how people talk about pleasure, I focus on the mechanisms directing the experience. This shift in thinking, influenced by a sociology of attachment, follows a similar trajectory to that recorded by Schwarz (2013) in regard to the sociological study of taste.

Influenced by the 'linguistic turn' and pulling away from an account of pleasure as a learnt practice (as exemplified in Becker's classic account), sociologists considering pleasure in relation to drug use have tended to study it in terms of how it gets discussed and known. For example, Coveney and Bunton (2003) distinguish four typologies of pleasure: carnal, disciplined, ascetic and ecstatic. But, like with 'taste', as seen in Schwarz's (2013) paper, there has been growing frustrations with an epistemological focus on the production of knowledge in a way that has underplayed how experiences are made in practice. Therefore, following the 'material turn' that has emerged over the last ten years or so in the drug field, much influenced by Gomart and Hennion's (1999) original paper, I attend here to the sociomaterial mechanisms of pleasure, and the techno-corporeal work involved in making oneself available to it.

However, this is a slightly different argument to some of the flatter ontologies taken in earlier accounts of the drug-using event, which, in perhaps an overzealous swing away from the human, have started to overlook the role of human bodies and processes and their uniquely intracorporeal qualities. As astutely observed by Bøhling, this

> might also be a result of Latour's methodological advice (2000; 2005a) only to describe the actions of directly observable social phenomena,

which, as some scholars point out (Krarup and Blok, 2011), may have created a kind of ontological bias towards the 'hard' (and nonhuman) actants (observable in spaces of consumption).

(2014: 364)

Instead, here, I look at the role of participants to collectively direct their bodies. That is, I focus on the mediation practices – the work. This is similar to Bøhling's account of modulation, where, drawing from Gabriel Tarde, he looks at how affective spaces get modulated in a nightclub. That is, how various non-human and human bodies 'generated emotional, sensorial and bodily energies that moved through, related and transformed the nightclub assemblage' (2014: 384). This more agentic account starts to make even more sense when we think about the fragile connections that I have observed as also partial connections – never subject/object, active/passive, but always somewhere in between. 'Partial connections', in Haraway's use of the term, are used in relation to the cyborg as 'a hybrid of machine and organism' (Haraway, 1991a: 149). Rather than the subject being whole – the basis of identity politics – one is only ever partially connected. Subjectivities or ontologies more generally are actively held together. But this means there is always room for them to be made differently. Taken up in Annemarie Mol's (2002) work, via Marilyn Strathern (1991), on atherosclerosis, the body is constituted differently through different practices, the body is therefore multiple and only ever partial – 'more than one and less than many'.

Consequently, the pleasure assemblage was only ever partial, and keeping these connections together ('keeping the glass upright') was an active part of participants' lives. Whilst I am by no means suggesting a return to the 're-lata' (Barad, 2007) individual agent, I am nonetheless suggesting there is an agentic force of collaboratively directing bodies towards or 'making oneself available' to pleasure, which is perhaps more agentic than other materialist turns. Hence, in returning to the classic text by Gomart and Hennion, I am continually surprised by how forward-thinking it was. For example, note how, even if unintentional, 'construction' is used rather than social construction in saying:

> This is not a critique of the 'construction' of the subject. Rather, it is an attempt to offer an alternative account of the ways in which subjects may be seized, *impassioned* and swept away. How to describe the devices by which amateurs (in the widest sense) are able to put their passion into practice?
>
> (Gomart and Hennion, 1999: 220–21, my emphasis)

Hennion's (2001; 2007; with Gomart, 1999) concept of the amateur is particularly useful for this study in considering how these attachments get negotiated – 'how the devices by which amateurs (in the widest sense) are able to use to put their passion into practice?' (Gomart and Hennion, 1999: 221). Within this approach, it is the attachments that make the subject experience rather than the subject making the attachments: 'he develops a disposition' through this relationality. In citing Hennion et al.'s (2000) work, a scholar from a completely different field of study, Meyer, notes:

> It is through the study of (partial) connectivities, that one can get a better grasp of the identities, practices, and roles of amateurs. This means considering amateurism not as an essence, but as relationally defined through *fragile* connections and demarcations. It means examining the relational complex, based upon objects, places, and collectives that *produces* the amateur.
>
> (2008: 49, original emphasis)

This does something very different to Bourdieu's practice theory (the subject of Hennion's critique), and Becker's theory of pleasure as a social accomplishment – 'to suggest instead that action is an unanticipated gift from the "dispositif"' (Gomart and Hennion, 1999: 222).

'A gift' seems to be much more applicable than Becker's idea of drugs' pleasures being accomplished through social interaction: 'He has learned, in short, to answer "Yes" to the question: "Is it fun?"' (1953: 243). The 'success' of injecting here, even if participants did everything that was required, often seemed to be out of their hands. What seemed clear is that being able to say 'yes' or 'no' was not so much when the participants said 'yes' or 'no' – in fact, Lucy was repeatedly saying 'yes', whilst Simon, in regard to the dangers, was saying 'no' – but it was the assemblage, a shared sense of control that prevailed. Simon describes this agency as 'it just happens', which echoes Gomart and Hennion's (1999) argument that drug consumption is not a matter of *doing* something but making something *happen* (getting 'moved' or 'impassioned'). But this is perhaps more than an accumulative effect of traceable actants. A gift accounts for something more – there is an extra quality, even a more than human quality – there is a sense of the world giving back. This resonates with Barad's (2007) idea that 'things don't just come out any way we'd like them to, there is a sense in which "the world kicks back"' (2007: 215).

In a similar way that Schwarz (2013) uses Hennion (2003; 2007) and Gomart and Hennion (1999) to think about the ways art lovers 'direct their bodies towards art works', I use this frame to think about what participants did or underwent to prepare their bodies for injecting drugs in a way that could enact pleasure – to 'make something happen' (Gomart and Hennion, 1999). I will attend to two types of work that came out particularly strongly in my research regarding how participants made themselves available to the pleasure assemblage: finding a vein and negotiating tolerance.

There was extensive work carried out around preparing the body for an injection. The practices highlight just how active this pursuit was and the importance of everything being in the right place for the assemblage to work, for pleasure to be produced. Again, with the slightest shift, this could all change – the world could kick back. Some of these practices, which I look at here, were around raising blood pressure – for example, 'warming up', cycling, eating, drinking alcohol, washing-up – relaxing (with Valium and alcohol), locating a vein and then getting a needle to stay in the blood vessel long enough for the injection to work.

Simon talks about how the pleasures of heroin – what he describes in relation to his 'pre-heroin' days as the feeling of 'coming home having done something really good at work or done something that's made you feel really good about yourself' – have started to become disrupted or put at risk by 'the difficulty of finding somewhere' (the effects of which are discussed further below). Negotiating these difficulties, Simon describes the carefully attuned, sensorial practices required to make the connections work:

> Now, what I tend to do. It has to be when I'm... it'd have to be in the evening. I will have to have eaten. I'd have to have had a few drinks to relax me, definitely will have had to have eaten. I mean, you know, I used to do it in the morning before I'd even woken up kind of thing, you know what I mean, so I would have had no blood pressure what so ever. But because my veins were so good it would still work. Now that, no way, it has to be the whole thing of hot water, do the washing up, make sure I've eaten and you can see the little tiny marks. So what it is now, is that I'll see a tiny little one, or I'll just do it by feeling, you just rub very, very, very gently, rubbing your hand around like that (shows me how he delicately rubs his hand), and I'll just feel something that gives a little bit and I know that's a vein.

For Simon, the injecting assemblage had become so fragile that he now only takes the risk once a month. I have looked already at how Valium helps, but here he talks more explicitly about other embodied techniques: 'I'd have to have a few drinks to relax me', 'definitely will have to have eaten', do 'the whole thing of hot water, do the washing up', see 'the little tiny marks' and feel for when something 'gives a little', and below he also describes having to be in a particular 'frame of mind':

> Well what would happen is, if I haven't done it for quite a while and I've been smoking [heroin] instead and haven't been using that much, I'll be in that frame of mind, something will happen, I'll be really pissed off, or I really want a good night sleep or and, it's just this really certain frame of mind, and I'll think I'm just going to have a hit now, I'm just going

to have it, and my veins are really up and it's worked and ... but then I'll leave it a while, because it's that satisfactory that it's worked, I don't want to push it.

The time of day and when he had already had something to smoke was also crucial for relaxing his body:

I couldn't stand the messing about, so that's why it's now becoming in the evening, when I've already had lots to smoke, and I'm quite relaxed, and I'm, I can find a hit, and it'll be okay, every now and again.

Conversely, for Lucy, being 'active' was key, but still nothing could guarantee 'success':

the places where usually work just didn't work for me and if I was busy, active, the veins would come up in my hand and that's where it'd be successful. But my hands would just work or they wouldn't work.

Lucy talked about washing-up to raise veins and Tom talked about cycling 'flat out' to increase his blood pressure. But the stigma of continuing to inject even though they found it incredibly hard was always in the background, and sometimes made it a difficult subject to discuss. For example, Tom says 'at the moment I'm desperate' but then quickly corrects himself to say 'I'm lucky to find anything'. The politics of continuing to inject despite the difficulty and harms caused seemed to be particularly linked to the presence of blood, which I discuss further below.

An increased physical tolerance to participants' preferred substances required added negotiation and embodied techniques to stabilise the assemblage in a way that could enact pleasure. Tolerance was often expressed as a source of great frustration for participants:

Taking crack or coke and then taking heroin, that's what it does, one minute they are up there and the next, all of a sudden, they come crashing down and the heroin kicks in – they are all falling over. That's why we see a lot of users they wake up and boom, fall down. *I would love to feel like that for 10 minutes, but I can't. Your tolerance gets to a stage.*

(Carlos)

As one's tolerance (of heroin, in particular) grew, participants often had to take additional preparatory steps to be 'moved' by the 'dispositif'.

For me to gouch, I would have to, errr, not use for a week or something like that, then your body just like ain't used to the heroin so like, if you get a decent bit, then you will gouch from it, but that's like, that's only like if you're sitting there relaxed.

(Carlos)

Participants said how they often had to change the quantity and ratio of water to heroin:

I'd have to make sure that the quantity that I'm putting in there is much darker and bigger to make it work.

(Jim)

So we might split this in half but if I really wanted to have a nice time, I'd have the lot. But we often, at least to get properly stoned, we need at least one each.

(Lucy)

For Carlos, it's not just a matter of tolerance but physical dependency, so in the morning, when there are less opiates in his system, he had to increase the quantity of the drug:

For example, in the morning, if I only do 1:1 [1 £10 bag of heroin: 1 £10 bag of crack] I feel it for a minute or two and then, it goes the same, that's why I usually do 2:1 in the morning and less liquid. For example, now, today, after 4/5 [injections of 'speedballs'], I use more liquid, more diluted so it gets a bit weaker, but in the morning, I will be 2:1 [heroin: crack] and I will put 60mls of water, so it's more strong.

For others, tolerance to the substance required additional alcohol and other drugs (also considered previously in terms of Valium). Jim says how now, even when he has a 'speedball', the 'niggling negative thoughts' do not subside. Clarifying on this, I ask 'so even when you're experiencing the high, you can still get some [negative thoughts]?' and Jim replies: 'Yeah, so now [...] that's why I'll have a drink on top of it, I'll have stuff on top of it, there's just not enough drugs in the world'.

Regardless of how much he tries to negotiate or mediate his 'tolerance' – 'there's just not enough drugs in the world' – pleasure as a particular enactment (devoid of other negative affects) has been lost. This points to where a relational, ANT-influenced account may be limited, and suggests that rather than each encounter starting anew, they, from a Deleuzian perspective, never end. Where Latourian accounts are more specifically and practically focussed in the methodology of close observation, a more abstract account can help to elucidate the less tangible. For example, Latour seems to, at least in relation to the experiment, suggest that there is an end to the event, 'a conclusion': 'no event can be accounted for by a list of the elements that entered the situation *before* its conclusion' (1999b: 126, original emphasis). Tolerance, on the other hand, speaks to a residual affect – an invisible excess – in which it is part of an ongoing event. I will return to this theme in Chapter 5 in terms of habit.

So far in this chapter, I have shown how pleasure is reliant on the successful coming together of a network of interacting human and non-human bodies and forces in the injecting event, and the active techno-corporeal work involved in making oneself available to these fragile connections. It is clear then, to quote Mol, 'undergoing, then, as in "undergoing pleasure" does not mean doing nothing at all' (2010: 257). Therefore, the next section explores participants' embodied experiences of this 'success' and how the assemblage gets felt. However, to reiterate, this is a fragile matter, so for many participants, just as easily as it comes together, it can also slip or 'drop' (to use Lucy's analogy) producing much more negative a/effects.

'Success!'

This section explores what happens when the injecting assemblage comes together 'successfully': when the metaphorical glass has been carefully steadied and that precious sip taken. As we have seen, enacting this 'success', as Lucy calls it, is a complicated affair and the modalities of feelings produced are no less complex. 'Success', rather than, say, 'rush', is an interesting choice of words because it accounts for a sense of pleasure and remedy at the same time, where the two cannot be separated. So, when participants talked about the pleasures of their injecting, it was often not purely active, but also reactive to a state of discomfort, stress or pain. Again, this points to the Deleuzian notion that connections in the event are not made anew but are ongoing. 'The hit' also simultaneously describes the process of injecting or 'hitting up' – the needle piercing the skin's surface to enter a vein – whilst also accounting for the embodied experience of the effect – the sense of heroin 'hitting' the body, or what one participant called 'hitting the spot' – in which the two almost seem synonymous. 'It's the feeling of putting it in, from getting in the vein, to pushing it in, it's that feeling, that it's instant', says Lucy. The needle, drug and body are entwined in this embodied 'success'.

Many multisensorial and visceral terms were used to explain the experience of when these complex assemblages of bodies aligned to enact pleasure, including feeling 'wrapped in cotton cool', 'glowing', 'waves', 'warm', 'buzzing', 'better than sex', 'an immense feeling', 'you just feel good' and 'all your problems go'. To accentuate this further, Ajay says:

> It's an immense feeling of just, I dunno, you just feel good innit, you just feel nice, yeah, and obviously, the reason why you keep on going back to it is because you like that feeling.

Grigor, in emphasising how embodied the experience is, re-enacts the feeling:

> It's coming from the whole of your body and it's like tingling, shaking as well, like a kind of shaking, ohh, ohh (acts out a pleasurable shivering motion), shivering.

The throat and taste, in particular, were central to this feeling:

> When I get a vein, I get that instant feeling and umm something like, your throat goes warm and it's just, it's just nice.
>
> (Grigor)

To a similar effect, Carlos also says:

> Oh yeah, you feel it in the throat. Ahh, you get the taste. As soon as you get the injection, you feel the taste, it's immediate. The same with cocaine as well.

These descriptions share commonalities with Vitellone's (2003b) work on the 'rush', which showcases the syringe to be very much part of the materialisation of the techno-corporeal event ('rush'). However, perhaps what is missing from Gomart and Hennion's (1999) account of drug users' pleasures and Vitellone's (2003b) account of the 'rush' is a reflection on dependency. Where the 'event' has been traced in drug research, this has also mainly been in 'recreational' settings (e.g. Bøhling, 2014; Dilkes-Frayne, 2014; Duff, 2012; Farrugia, 2015; Race, 2014), so, again, dependency is rarely present. For many of my informants, the injecting event did more than enact pleasure, but also provided relief from painful withdrawal symptoms, discomfort or/and stress. For example, for Simon, there was a strong sense that the relief and rush from injecting heroin were one of the same:

> It's just incredible, it's just an instant feeling of, feeling just like (takes a massive inhale and exhale of air – wooohhh), all that stuff [withdrawal symptoms] [see Figure A.2] goes and all the various types of, all the various different conditions, symptoms, are gone, gone… It's like nothing else does it, and that's why I think you do become, there is a sort of, kind of, a love affair, that starts to happen, because there is no other medicine in the world that does that, I can't [pause] I try to [pause] I've spent years trying to explain to people…

But, furthermore, there was also a feeling of relief in the assemblage working, beyond the causal 'effect' of the drug assemblage, that is, in its *working*, rather than a product of it working. Lucy, for example, refers to a feeling of 'winning the lottery' not in terms of the pleasure resulting from the injection working but in the very fact that it worked: 'I've damaged these veins so badly but I've had success, like a friend said to me, oh you sound happy and I said "I found a vein that works again" so that was like winning the lottery'.

For Tom, the sense of relief from the injection working is extended further. He feels this relief most starkly in relation to the even wider completion of the scoring process. On his body map, he draws a smile and I ask:

FD: So, you're smiling because you're happy?
TOM: Yeah
FD: Anything else? ... just because you're high?
TOM: Yeah, basically, it's always a *relief* when you err..., do you know what I mean, I hate, I absolutely hate scoring drugs, I loathe it, I, years ago, when I was making good money selling [products] at Christmas I used to pay a dodgy guy who used to hang out in the corner in [south London] to go and score for me, I'd give him like 50 quid and say look go and get us three and I'll buy you one or two and pay him 10, 20 quid just to pick up for him cos I hate hanging around council estates or stairwells or d'you know what I mean. Just hanging out waiting for some fucking prick to turn up and take my money off me (sigh) so I absolutely loathe scoring, and it's always stressful, and you're always on the lookout for the police and then you've got to worry about popping things in your mouth and just hoping that you get back before you get stopped and have to swallow them and blahblahblah...
...But as soon as I've actually found a vein, got the hit and it's in, no lumps or bumps and you can feel it come on then it's just a feeling of relief, that's a feeling of relief, do you know what I mean, you can just relax, chill out.

The hit, for Tom, encompasses a 'feeling of relief' (rather than rush), which takes the injecting assemblage beyond the needle-substance-nervous system, into the social and legal status of drugs. The assemblage here extends to the illegality of heroin which causes Tom a great deal of stress in terms of the potentiality of getting arrested ('look out for the police'), the dislike of the areas that he is forced to go to ('I hate hanging around council estates'), and the people he has to meet and pay ('some fucking prick'), which means that being able to 'get a hit' was as much about relief from that situation as it was about the pleasure it could bring. In fact, he is quite dismissive of the way people describe this pleasure – 'it's like being wrapped in cotton wool or whatever they say'. The success of the scoring is part of the 'hit' *working* – 'as soon as I've actually found a vein, and it's in' – which, taken together, takes the pleasurable feeling well beyond the causal effect of the drug.

But, a sense of this 'relief' being beyond his control is again driven home:

> ...And quite often, the one, the hit that you do the first, the first one, if you've been out all day trying to make your money or whatever, the first one, when you're really needing to., tends to be the one that you struggle to find a vein. If I've cycled like a maniac and my blood's flowing really fast through the body and all that, and my veins should be pumping, that tends to be the hardest one to find. The second one, when you've already had a hit, and you're already quite chilled out, tends to be the one when you get it straight off (clicks his fingers to show the fast speed of it).

In this passage, like many above (e.g. the way Valium relaxes the body), Tom is actively engaged in sociomaterial practices and techniques of opening himself up to the full effect of the rush-relief. But what became obvious, in a similar way to 'tolerance', is that, for some, this desired openness or receptiveness (what I have considered as an active-passivity) was getting harder to achieve. For instance, and in explicit reference to the 'ritual' (process) rather than the causal effect, instead of being able to enjoy the hit, Lucy wanted another one straight away:

> But that *ritual*, even if we've been successful, what's so weird, that because you've had the feeling of that working and that's been enjoyable, even though you're stoned, you want to do it again quite soon. So 'want again, because I enjoyed that' (she writes on the body map). And it's just after long term use, so long term use, success is... cos you're just thinking wow it's worked, I've damaged these veins so badly but I've had success.

Several other participants also talked about this need to inject again. As I have said, this repetition is largely overlooked in Gomart and Hennion's study and in other ANT-influenced studies of the drug-using event. Amongst participants here it seemed that a state of passivity was only momentarily possible or not even. Many participants, therefore, talked about their dissatisfaction with the quality of the drugs and their frustrations at not being able to achieve the same high as they once could.

> So even though I'm sort of feeling the high, I'm already disappointed... And like I said, disappointed with myself, and I'm so disappointed in drugs, they're not good enough, *they're not doing what they're meant to.* I feel cheated because I've taken the drugs and what they used to do to me they don't do no more.
>
> (Jim)

For Jim, the connections were simply not working – he was failing to be 'impassioned'. Similarly, Dimitri says: 'I haven't had a proper gouch for ages'.

Many participants seemed to be experiencing some sort of failure in not being able to achieve pleasure, and, in particular, the pleasure achieved by 'beginners' (especially in regard to heroin) was widely missed – what participants often phrased as 'chasing the high'.

Although, as stated above, active work was done to negate and mediate 'tolerance' in opening oneself up to the passivity necessary to be overcome by pleasure, in some cases this was not possible, but in others it was not even desired. For instance, 'gouching' – what Simon calls 'the ultimate goal of every "junkie"' – was often seen as controllable and dependent on what one was doing, the time of day, the dose and the environment (including the chair, which is seen in both Reggie's [above] and Gwen's body map [see Figure A.1):

> If you're sitting there relaxed, but, like, if you're doing things and everything, it doesn't... the gouching part is only if you are sitting there and you're relaxed. If you're up doing something, it's not like it will make you sit there and gouch, it doesn't do it like that, it depends like what you're doing.
>
> (Vicki)

> [How long the gouching lasts] depends on the dose, a gouch could last, it depends, an hour, it could last half an hour, it depends when you want to wake up out of it.
>
> (Ajay)

> [I would be gouching for] an hour, two hours, it depends. It depends on how much I take... depends on the environment that I'm in, cos if I'm with people in a crack house, I don't really know them and that, then I can't relax in there.
>
> (Reggie)

And, for Grigor, the controllability of the 'gouch' from injecting not only made it more efficient ('it goes on a lot longer'), but also made it more pleasurable (you can 'postpone it until you're ready'):

> you can kind of postpone the hit when you inject, you can feel the initial buzz but the gouching as well, *which most uses like*, you can kind of, you know, *postpone* it until you're ready and sit down and then you can kind of chill into it. But with smoking, it's there and done and gone, you know, you're not gonna feel like that again until you get more gear... With injecting, you know, it goes on a lot longer

For me, this reintroduces an idea of 'control' as discussed in the Introduction through Poulsen's (2015) and Weinberg's (2013) very different post-human accounts. Poulsen (2015) uses Barad's agential realism to argue that drug enactments cannot be controlled by the user, whilst Weinberg (2013) uses Latour's theory of the body to reinvigorate a loss of self-control as a set of learnt practices and embodied sensitivities, which he sees to be at the heart of addiction. Responding to Weinberg's (2013) call to re-engage with control, albeit a loss of self-control, I consider the injecting assemblage as an event which demonstrates shared control (Dennis, 2016; Poulsen, 2015). Like Poulsen, 'agency is understood to be shaped by the intra-actions that make up a phenomenon' (2015: 13). That is, the 'control' that participants expressed over their drug practices was always in connection to others, human and non-human.

> Do we hold something or does something hold onto us? Beyond such reciprocity, which would remain profoundly dualist, the connections to the diverse natures in which we are entangled, that hold us and which hold us together, call for redistribution of agency, deployed in the interlacing of ins and outs where every connection does something, but where none is sufficient on its own.
>
> (Hennion, 2012)

In fact, for some, pleasure was found in harnessing the potentiality of the energy that drug assemblages could produce, but interestingly this happened in very political ways. In particular, the 'rush' for many women got enacted and, dare I say, enjoyed in an acutely gendered way.

> I'd feel more likely to clean [...] you feel like you want to do stuff, otherwise, you know, you don't do anything.
>
> (Gwen)

> Gosh, yeah. Sometimes, particularly with crack, give me a bag of crack and I can turn my flat into a show home. Whizz around with the hoover.
>
> (Suzy)

> But heroin is one of those drugs, if you don't do it daily, if it's recreational, it can actually make you ... I used to get up and clean my house in the middle of the night.
>
> (Nadiya)

> I start doing housework, clean my house, everything, it gives me energy at first, if you take more you start to 'gouch' out but at first I'll be cleaning my house.
>
> (Meg)

Interestingly, none of the male participants referred to the 'buzz' in relation to cleaning. The way drug effects get felt is therefore already part of something bigger. Far from a drug-body interaction, with neurochemicals literally dictating the 'path' (neurological pathways), heteronormative ideas of what it is to be a woman were already party to the mix. There is a politics to affects (such as pleasure) and feelings that otherwise get left out. How the hit gets felt is again based on sociomaterial entanglements. It is in this way that Barad discusses intra-actions – the body and discourses do not interact, but are already one of the same.

Where an actor-network approach has been criticised for lacking the tools to deal with issues of power and inequality (Restivo, 2005; 2011; Rudy and Gareau, 2005), a politics of affect is better equipped. An affective politics works to determine ways of becoming. Where the body is defined through its ability to affect and be affected (always in relation), it can become contained in some connections, which constrain these affective powers. For example, bodies stratified by gendered structures that stereotype women in terms of roles and responsibilities (seen in urges to clean) prevent other ways of becoming. In post-structural phenomenology, most notably in feminist traditions (Ahmed, 2004; Del Busso and Reavey, 2013; Fraser et al., 2014: 13), how we come to feel is affected by our encounters with bodies that capacitate these feeling. Most explicitly in regard to drugs and pleasure, Race (2009) considers how a politics of pleasure constrains queer ways of becoming. According to Massumi (2015), the difference between structuralist and post-structuralist accounts is that the latter is intrinsically more hopeful, that is, every encounter brings the potential to do something new. A central part of academic practice is therefore to produce better affects – a theme I return to in the book's conclusion.

To sum up, this section has attended to some of the ways pleasure materialises as rush-relief, which goes beyond other techno-corporeal accounts of the drug event that tend to focus on the rush. That is, it is reactive as well as active, respondent to affects as well as able to make new ones. But what if the pleasure assemblage shifts – what if the metaphorical glass drops?

The glass drops: slipping assemblages

Lucy points out that missing a hit or 'dropping the glass' is more than a lack of 'success' (rush-relief), but could also result in extreme pain: 'but my god when you have a miss, electric shocks can happen, you can hit capillaries, a nerve, the abscesses explode…'. Furthermore, the connections involved in bringing this assemblage together in a pleasurable way were made all the more fragile by this potentialised pain. Therefore, accounts of 'success' were often juxtaposed against such accounts of failure.

Participants talked about several situations of the injecting event 'going wrong'. Telling me about how he once hit an artery, Ed says:

> I've ended up on my knee caps, it really hurt, it killed me, I was on my knees, like urrhh (making crying out noises), it really hurt, I was in a lot

of pain, a big electric shock it was, it really hurt, I've never had a pain like it, it killed me.

Lucy recounts getting an abscess, which led to her hand 'ballooning' to the point that she could not get her rings off and risked losing a finger:

> I've had horrible abscesses. The worse one was a complete electric shock because you're pushing in somewhere nowhere near a vein, it's right on a nerve ending and a capillary, which is a tiny thing that can't cope and it's exploding it and it was like the most horrible electric shock in my hand, and my hand looked like a balloon. And it had, I had rings on, so when I went to the ambulance. They had to cut the rings off quick because they said I was going to lose circulation and I had my hand up here and it was like a giant balloon, like a dummy hand, it was full of fluid.

Although abscesses and hitting an artery were extremely painful, it was often the 'dirty hit' that was most feared. Its storied presence was foreboding for those that had not experienced it, which loomed over each injection. The exact cause of a 'dirty hit' was unknown but felt by participants to be caused by dirt, bacteria or a cutting agent entering the injection solution. Gwen explains:

> A dirty hit, could be, you get someone to inject for you and they've got dirty hands, there could be something nasty in the gear and you haven't done it proper, *if you're not careful* with a clean needle and a clean swab, the dirt gets into it... They call it a dirty hit, it could be a cut in it, and it's going into the needle.

The pain caused by a dirty hit is known amongst injectors to be so excruciating that Gwen says:

> If I get a dirty hit, I'll stop [...] it'll put me off it forever, luckily I've never had one, but I've seen people do it, they shake, they go into immediate withdrawal, they shake, start throwing up, people are crying, if that happens to me, I'm never doing it again.

Sue also comments on the extremity of the discomfort:

> I've had a dirty hit and it's horrible. I actually did it down [...] with this guy, down this alley, he got a can of coke, the top of it, turned it upside down and we washed it in that, and we both got a dirty hit and I was ill the whole day, cos you know you get a bit of dust in the needle. You're so ill, even if you take more heroin it takes time to get out your system, it's a horrible feeling, you know, you're aching like made, really bad in

my legs and you have to keep on doing that (shakes her legs out) because you feel like you're going to have a fit.

The dirty hit is one of many effects that can emerge if the attachments shift, and hence Gwen stresses the importance of being 'careful', as introducing a tiny bit of dirt into the injecting assemblage could result in something so painful that, for Gwen, at least, it would put her off injecting for good.

Participants also spoke of the stress and emotional pain of 'the hit' not working, again, producing affects beyond a lack of pleasure. The labour-intensive process of searching for and piercing a viable vein, large enough to hold a needle steady to draw back some blood and inject the solution, without going through the other side, could sometimes last for several hours. If too much air entered the mix, and blood coagulated in the needle, it could render the mixture untenable, causing huge distress. To this effect, Simon states:

> I was sometimes losing the entire lot, it started to coagulate, and you'd have to just chuck it away, and that would probably mean chucking it against the wall in fury... And you know, you look down at your arms and all your body and you're just *covered in blood*, you know, you're covered in it, and there's no, none of this (points to the picture of him enjoying the effects of heroin [see Figure A.2]), and you're still feeling like this (points to the picture of him before he's used), but *you're just covered in blood*.

A similar sense of not only fury, but also disgust was depicted by Jim:

> And I just won't just give up on it. I'm just determined I'm gonna get the vein. And in the end it's just turned, it's got too clotted with blood that I've just lost it (got really angry)... And then I've got to go out and try and get it all over again. And like really it's quite *filthy* to look at.

Here, I want to think about not only the presence of air in rendering the solution useless, but the role blood is playing, in particular, as an actant plugging into a whole new set of bodies and discourses with stratifying tendencies. The presence of blood is accentuated in Lucy's account: 'You know, and it just means blood, whatever happens there's going to be blood around...'. The politics of blood is well documented in accounts of racism (Ahmed, 2003), menstruation (Bobel, 2010; Laws, 1990) and homophobia (Eagles, 2015), but is less considered in prejudice towards injecting drug users. One notable exception is Harris's (2009) paper on injecting and hepatitis C stigma. Drawing on this paper and a paper written by Fraser and valentine (2006) on 'materialising blood' in relation to BDSM (bondage and domination, dominance and submission and sadomasochism), I want to look at what blood *does* in producing the failed, abject injecting event. Rather than signifying the failure of the injecting event, it seems to be doing more, in actively producing it, and other (unpleasant) affects.

In Fraser and valentine's (2006) paper, they use Barad (2003) to consider blood in BDSM not as a prior essence, but as a 'phenomenon', which materialises in different ways depending on its intra-action with discourse and matter. In becoming something new in these intra-actions, it also produces differences in meaning, identity (as both essence and non-essence) and ownership, and enacts pleasure. Drawing on this account in relation to abjection, blood changes and produces new affects. For Julia Kristeva, the abject is produced in breaking down the boundaries between one body and another. Using Kristeva's concept, Harris (2009) writes: 'the act of injecting can be seen to threaten order, in that it contravenes social demarcations between the exterior and interior of the body'. Bleeding is a transgressive point where these boundaries become blurred or contaminated. The injecting drug user as a figure who disrupts boundaries is a central theme in 'junkie literature' and film (Bowers, 2009), the 'heroin chic' genre of the 1990s (Malins, 2009) and media representations of town 'no-go zones' (Fitzgerald and Threadgold, 2004). Simon and Jim's accounts above stress the role of blood in producing the failed assemblage and abjection rather than pleasure: 'you're just left covered in blood'. Lucy also accounts for this failure using affective, abject terms, such as 'revolting', 'depressing', 'desperate' and 'ugly': 'it gets really depressing how revolting it gets, how desperate it gets to try and get a hit to work, it gets really ugly'.

In a similar way to Vitellone's (2010) account of the syringe, I consider blood as a politically affective object. Citing Ahmed (2004), Vitellone explains that

> it is not that an object might be inherently disgusting but rather that 'an object becomes disgusting through contact with other objects that have already, as it were, been designated as disgusting' [...] After AIDS, the injecting drug user has indeed come to signify contamination, disease, and disgust.
>
> (Vitellone, 2010: 875)

Like the syringe, I suggest that blood has become equally 'contaminated' through discursive connections. For example, contracting hepatitis C through the blood of another injector in the process of injecting is gravely more stigmatising than contracting it through blood products (Fraser, 2004; Fraser and Treloar, 2006; Harris, 2005; Harris and Rhodes, 2013b; Seear et al., 2010). Connecting with this blood, especially at its most disruptive, when a lot is outside the body, produces abjection. Almost echoing Kristeva's (1982) essay, *Powers of Horror*, Lucy says: 'it went back to a horror show again where it's just a case of not being able to find somewhere to go [...]

and it's just like a blood bath, *there's blood everywhere*. It's just, you know, depressing'.

There is a symbolic resonance in the blood beyond the moment and a discursive quality intra-acting with the material. This is seen in Jim's earlier statement in which he is clearly aware of a wider audience/gaze: 'really it's quite filthy to look at'. Where Fraser and valentine (2006) stress blood as a phenomenon that constantly changes in meaning and ownership, here, there is also a sense of permanence in blood's affective powers that appear to transcend events. To appropriate Vitellone's sentiment on the syringe, the blood of injecting drug users has already been 'designated disgusting'. For example, in continuing his explanation of the 'filthy' coagulated needle, Jim stresses the abjection in saying how he has also injected *Special Brew* (a substance embedded with stigma)[4] and puddle water. Blood seems to be both bringing affects and producing new ones in the injecting event. Participants' accounts suggest that whilst blood is getting made in its affectiveness, so too are particular feelings, emotions and even bodies. Put more concisely, blood (as discourse-matter) produces injecting events (as needle-drug-blood) that enact abjected states.

To return to Lucy's metaphor of the glass, the assemblage has shifted, and the techniques to raise a vein and relax the body have not worked. She cannot find a vein to use, and instead the skin is punctured, and, as she says above, 'blood is everywhere'. The pleasure assemblage has failed, the 'high' is not felt, and instead another assemblage gets made, where, in particular, the blood as an affectively politically charged substance, already in connection to other discursive-material bodies, produces an array of negative emotions and subjectivities. The fragility of the assemblage gets accentuated in the *difference* between it working and failing, what Lucy depicts in her body map as a '50/50' chance, between it being 'successful' – the high ('hehehe') – or 'the drama', where, like a typical television murder drama, there is blood everywhere.

> I mean, *the difference,* if it's successful, you're like 'hehehe' and like floating. But the drama if you have a miss, the anger and... *it's horrible.* .... there's this 50:50 if it's going to work, 50 heaven, 50 hell.

'The difference' in affects is more than a lack of pleasure (rush-relief), but an enactment of a whole new cascade of feelings and forces. Unsurprisingly, for Lucy, like others, this fragility was getting too much. Where some turned to femoral injecting, described as 'cleaner', 'quicker' and 'neater' (suggesting perhaps less blood), Lucy, and at least three other participants, turned to smoking. The attachments of the injecting assemblage, which meant that success could not be guaranteed, had become so brittle that they had opted to smoke as a more definite way of in-corporating (into the corpus/body) heroin or/and crack cocaine.

And then when I started injecting again, recently, I noticed that, how quickly the veins, how I'm struggling and they're not working and it goes back quickly to the, not having any success, going on for hours, feeling blinding, washing things to try and pump, get the veins up, pouring with sweat. The whole thing becomes horrible and even though you get somewhere, even that becomes more dominant in my head, the nightmare that I went through, so I think I'd rather just smoke it, and really get a lung full and get stoned, rather than have that nightmare.

(Lucy)

For Lucy, the pleasure assemblage is no longer coming together; most notably, the veins are not 'working'. And she says, talking yourself into a subcutaneous (as opposed to an intravenous) injection does not work: 'when you sort of have a miss, you know it hasn't quite worked but you try to *talk yourself into it*. Even though, you're really cross because of all the ritual and everything' – she expects more from her preparations – this is more than words alone can deal with, that is, talking herself into it is not going to be enough. Whilst this statement emphasises the importance of words and conscious narrativisation, it also stresses that they are not always enough. Perhaps, for Becker's participants, this would have worked (learning to answer 'yes'), but not here.

Once again, there is an overriding sense that the subject is just one of many actors in the injecting event. Although their skills and techniques are necessary in terms of nurturing the fragile connections and aiding the passivity necessary to be moved by pleasure, there is a sense that the relational whole will win out, which is beyond any*one's* control. Although this is seen most vividly in the accounts of those who are struggling with the injecting itself, especially Lucy, Jim, Tom and Simon, even those not struggling are dependent on these aligning relations: the timings, substances, quantities, routes, people around them, spaces, equipment, etc. Nowhere is this balancing more evident than in the case of the speedball. Therefore, for the remainder of this chapter, I will briefly turn to this pleasure assemblage *par excellence*.

Balancing the 'speedball': 'a different drug altogether'

With [...] pleasure, the effects are not exogenous variables, or automatic attributes of objects. They are the results of a corporeal practice, collective and instrumented, settled by methods that are discussed endlessly, oriented around the appropriate seizing upon of uncertain effects. It is for this reason that we prefer to speak of attachments.

Antoine Hennion, 2007: 109

In this final section, I turn specifically to the speedball as a particular kind of attachment, which exemplifies the fragile injecting assemblage and active-passive work of directing bodies towards pleasurable encounters. The 'speedball' is a simultaneous injection of heroin and crack cocaine loaded in the same syringe. Thirteen participants were currently injecting speed-balls although almost all had tried it. The speedball conjured up powerful thoughts and feelings, what several participants described as the 'best' and 'only' way to do it. Unique to the speedball was its ability to take the user both *up and down*:

> Oh, well, where I've done both, I've got the up and the down, it's like beam me up scotty and then wooooo, you know, a frizzle down, after the white [crack]. After the up, you get a frizzle down and you get the come down off the heroin.
>
> (Anita)

> You get a buzz from both of it, together. You get the initial, the high from the crack, then you get the mellow feeling from the brown [heroin], well that's what you should get but the brown's shit these days.
>
> (Crystal)

> The brown will relax you and make you sleepy and sedated, the cocaine will heighten your senses and you know, you get a rush from it [....] If you do them both together, initially you'll feel the cocaine first, for about 5 or 10 minutes, and then the brown will start to kick in after that, and as the cocaine starts to wear off, the brown will kick in and like, a lot of people just think it's a better way of doing it.
>
> (Mike)

Interestingly, the speedball was considered 'a different drug altogether': not a mixture of heroin and crack, but rather something that exceeded the two. In a powerful analogy, Carlos compares the speedball to drinking 'whiskey cola', which he says is not like drinking whiskey and cola, but something altogether different.

CARLOS: I tried many times just to do the white (crack) and then do the heroin, it doesn't work, it's like, it's a waste, you don't feel it.

FD: (picking-up on what others had said) It's not like crack and heroin, it creates something different?

CARLOS: Exactly. For example, if you drink Coke, you drink Coca-Cola, you drink it and it's a nice juicy drink, you add whiskey, whiskey cola, it's different, but if you drink only whiskey 'errgh', but then if you put cola in it, you drink well and it feels different and it's nice. For example, if I give you four or five drinks of just whiskey, you may drink one, and go 'no, no, I don't want no more' but if I add Coca-Cola with it, you'll drink the rest as whiskey cola, right.

> [...] like I said, as soon as you start doing speedball, it's difficult just doing one, I'm just doing heroin more and more because of the white, if I do just white, I don't feel it, so I taking brown more and more because of the white. If it wasn't for the white, I wouldn't even take brown.

FD: So there's something about the brown that helps the white work?

CARLOS: Yes, it kind of levels out. Just the white it's too crispy, you know, it's like, like I said, if you drink whiskey it's crispy to go down, but add cola and it's more soft, more swarve, it's the same thing.

Carlos explains that he tried to take heroin and then crack but it didn't 'work'. The feeling of taking them together is different from taking them separately.

Using a similar analogy to Carlos (albeit a different kind of coke), Jim thinks about how the speedball creates a 'different drug altogether'.

> You use them individually and it's not the same. This sort of creates a different drug all together. With alcohol and cocaine they reckon makes a different drug. If you sit in a pub and sniff Charlie [cocaine], won't be like someone who's just sniffed Charlie, and it won't be like someone who's just had a drink. The two make a different, once they're in you, they combine and make a different effect.

This excess resonates with a Deleuzian via Spinoza understanding of the event, which is always beyond a sum of its parts. The event changes things, there is no undoing, but just constant sensitising and adjusting. There is nothing prior to the event; rather, 'mixtures' are the primary unit.

> Mixtures in general determine the quantitative and qualitative states of affairs: the dimensions of an ensemble – the red of iron, the green of a tree. But what we mean by 'to grow', 'to diminish', 'to become red', 'to become green', 'to cut', and 'to be cut' etc, is something entirely different. These are no longer states of affairs – mixtures deep inside bodies – but incorporeal events at the surface which are the results of these mixtures. The tree 'greens'.
>
> (Deleuze, 1990: 5–6)

By using the infinitive form, Deleuze is distinguishing the event – 'greening' – from the tree and greenness. Therefore, as Stagoll puts it, 'the event is not a disruption of some continuous state, but rather the state is constituted by events "underlying" it that, when actualised, mark every moment of the state as a transformation' (2010: 90). Similarly, Mike talks about the speedball becoming 'a whole different drug':

> It's almost as if when you combine the two different drugs it turns into *a whole different drugs*, I think that's how people perceive it, and that's

how it makes you feel, it's like you combine the two and it turns into something totally new, *a new substance*, and that's, I think, how your body absorbs it, and that's how it feels.

Both Mike and Jim explicitly talk about how the substances combine with the body ('once they're in you'; 'that's how your body absorbs it'). They become with the body in a different way than they should outside the body. This requires a different type of knowing – an embodied knowing or attunement. Mike explains this in terms of 'your body knows'.

If you inject heroin on its own, you'll get a certain feeling, if you inject crack on its own, you'll get a certain feeling, but it's never going to be the same [...] It still won't feel the same, because you'll know, *your body knows* it's just cocaine and you don't get that same feeling, it's hard to describe, but it kind of softens the edges and it's not so full on.

The speedball is a matter of body-substance intra-action that goes beyond the mechanical system of pharmacokinetics. The body cannot be manipulated through a combination of the substances, so much so that for Mike they have to be taken together or not at all: 'I won't entertain one without the other. I just won't do it'. There is also a sense that once the attachments are known, they are harder to change. Dimitri explains:

For example, if for someone who's never speedball, they will spend the rest of their life just smoking heroin or smoking white in a pipe and then smoking heroin and that will be it. But from the first time they speedball, that's it, that's it, *it's a different buzz*, I tried many times just to do the white and then do the heroin, it doesn't work, it's like, it's a waste, you don't feel it.

Grigor alludes to this particular attunement with the speedball, which means he is moved towards having 'one after the other':

I started really injecting crack, so-called 'speedball' 7–9 months, close to a year, ago [...] but I've never been back. I can't do it not speedball. If it's not speedball it's something just happening really and I'm not happy at all. So as soon as I started doing the speedball, I like it so much, but it makes me do one after the other after the other.

For Grigor, if it's not a speedball, its 'just something happening'. The satisfaction is not there. Yes, he feels something, but it's not 'success'. Therefore, what constitutes 'success' (rush-relief) has shifted: injecting crack cocaine and heroin separately 'doesn't work' or, for Mike, 'you don't feel it'. But, rather than an addiction to the substances, there is an attunement with them and the feelings enacted in their intra-action. This is perhaps why some participants who attended a diamorphine clinic continued to speedball or 'piggy back' crack onto the diamorphine injection as those specific feelings they were *used to* (attuned to) were not *achieved*. Like with 'tolerance', there is something residual in the event. Deleuze's green tree cannot pull apart. This is not to suggest people cannot stop using speedballs, but to simply highlight the difficulty in this kind of intervention, and to suggest that a more caring and generative intervention might focus on making new connections rather than breaking old ones. That is, there are never de-attachments but just new attachments. This is discussed further in Chapter 5.

Conclusion

Through Lucy's metaphor of the tilting water glass, this chapter has highlighted the precariousness of the injecting event in enacting pleasure. The first section developed a conceptual shift from Becker's understanding of pleasure as a social accomplishment to pleasure as a relational achievement. Drawing on Gomart and Hennion's (1999) and Latour's (1999a) sociology of attachment, instead of identifying a single actor who seeks out pleasure, pleasure is dependent on a fragile assemblage of human and non-human bodies, beyond any*one*'s control. This assemblage was explored in terms of substances, paraphernalia and space-time. But in reading these fragile connections as partial connections (Haraway, 1991a), I considered the active work necessary in keeping them together and directing bodies towards them. This reinvigorates the human and agentic in the more-than-human, where other turns to matter have tended to focus on the non-human. Pleasure required an active-passivity, similar to that seen in Hennion's (2001; 2007) work on 'taste'. But as this passivity required an openness to being taken by the assemblage, it could also take bodies in the wrong direction. Whilst there were techno-corporeal techniques to direct these bodies, such as stimulating the circulatory system, carefully locating an injection sight and negotiating tolerance, essentially it was the assemblage that won out.

It is perhaps no surprise then that, unlike previous studies, which have focussed on the rush, pleasure got felt here both as relief – at the assemblage working – and as rush. To further stress this relief, participants often compared the pleasure against the pain of failure – 'the difference'. With the slightest shift, for example, in making contact with a nerve ending or the introduction of dirt, bacteria or a cutting agent into the injecting solution, excruciating pain could erupt. But more than pain or a lack of pleasure, failure often got enacted as abjection. Here, I paid particular attention to the affective properties of blood as (already) affected and affecting in producing these subjectivities. Again, this emphasises a residual charge to the event, which supports a Deleuzian understanding of the event that has never ended. The final section attended to the speedball as a bodily attachment which stresses pleasure as a relational achievement, but also highlights the residual attunements that need to be taken seriously.

This chapter has shown how participants moved between activity and passivity, but what has become clear in this research, which was absent from Gomart and Hennion's (1999) seminal work and alcohol and other drugs (AOD) studies that have tended to focus on the rush of the event, is that this passivity has become harder and harder to reach, to the point that, for some, pleasure was only ever fleeting or had vanished entirely. Some participants were rarely overcome in perhaps the way they might have liked. Largely due to a focus on 'recreational' drugs, but also a certain post-structuralist interest in production and change over stasis, recent AOD studies of the event have tended to neglect the residual and repetitive affects that charge an atmosphere, which, for some participants, prevented the passivity required to become impassioned. But also, some participants, as seen in the way 'gouching' was managed, did not even desire this passivity to be 'swept away', and in this, the injecting event, quite drastically, seemed to become about something else. Taking this theme up in the next chapter, I look at how the injecting event, for some, had become about one of life's more fundamental tasks described as 'keeping oneself together' or 'becoming normal'. In this sense, the tilting glass of water becomes analogous for something even more *vital*.

Notes

1 I have since seen 'relational achievement' to be a phrase used by Law (1991: 166) in regard to how categories that appear natural are actively sustained, and more recently by Duff (2012) in relation to drug consumption. Here, it is used very much based on participants' accounts of relational 'success'.
2 Participants in this study tended to use the term needle rather than syringe.
3 This was part of a trial where people were given injectable diamorphine to administer under clinical supervision.
4 Special Brew is a high percentage beer, which is often associated with people who drink on the street.

Chapter 4

Living bodies

Vital becomings: becoming-normal, -other and -blocked *with* drugs

One does not hang together as a matter of course: keeping oneself together is something the embodied person needs to *do*. The person who fails to do so dies.

Annemarie Mol and John Law, 2004: 43

A lot of people want the up, the buzz as well, as lots of people go to work, working, living relatively normal lives, y'know, they have things to keep together, other lives to pretend to lead and stuff and cover up.

Vicki, 54 years old, injects diamorphine

You're not getting stoned no more, you're getting it to do normal things.

Mya, 52 years old, injects diamorphine

Where the last chapter was concerned with how the drug assemblage comes together to achieve success as a rush-relief, that is, the ways bodies become in pleasurable ways, here, I look at how the drug assemblage was enacted in less experimental (for visceral feelings), but yet perhaps more *vital* (for life) ways, in becoming 'normal' and 'other'. These vital becomings follow a Deleuzian notion of desire, in which life is not something given ('being'), but is the force that moves singularities into being, in which 'humans' are in a constant state of flux. In distinguishing the difference between desire and pleasure, and his preference for the former – 'I can barely stand the word pleasure' – Deleuze states:

For me, desire includes no lack; it is also not a natural given. Desire is wholly a part of a functioning heterogeneous assemblage. It is a process, as opposed to a structure or a genesis. It is an affect, as opposed to a feeling. It is heccity – the individual singularity of a day, a season, a life. As opposed to a subjectivity, it is an event, not a thing or a person. Above all it implies the constitution of a field of immanence or a body-without-organs, which is only defined by zones of intensity, thresholds, degrees and fluxes. This body is as biological as it is collective and political. It is on this body that assemblages are made and come apart, and this body-without-organs is what bears the offshoots of deterritorialisation of assemblages or flight lines.

(Deleuze, 1977: 130)

For Deleuze, desire is what moves us through life and therefore is inherently productive and should not be confused with lack. Desire is the foundational force by which bodies are produced in relation to other bodies. As Colebrook encapsulates, 'it is the productive process of life that produces organisms and selves' (2002: xii). As such, Deleuze, unlike Michel Foucault, would rather talk about desire than pleasure:

> I cannot give any positive value to pleasure because pleasure seems to interrupt the immanent process of desire. Pleasure seems to me to be on the side of strata and organisation; and in the same breath desire is presented as inwardly submitting to the law and outwardly regulated by pleasures. In both cases, there is a negation of the field of immanence proper to desire.
>
> (Deleuze, 1977: 20)

Bodies are 'desiring machines' (Deleuze and Guattari, 1987), that is, they are always in connection to other bodies and gain their power (and a lack of it) from these connections. A concept of desire helps to make sense of participants' accounts where drugs were about more than pleasure or pain relief (however broadly conceived) but becoming-normal and -other. Illicit drugs, rather than being inherently counter or destructive to life (in dominant ways of thinking about their misuse and addictive nature), were, for some, actively involved in preserving life – in keeping the body together and enacting human agency or what Sandra identifies, in her body map (Figure 4.1), as 'functioning for the rest of the day', 'shopping' and 'daily life'. The body, as a becoming of bodies (which can include drugs), must be actively held together (Mol, 1999; 2002; Mol and Law, 2004). This radically de-pathologises drug use by disrupting current ideas of life and 'the body' that rely on the binaries of inner/outer, self/other and human/non-human. It takes seriously the productive (life-fulfilling) work that, for many participants, both licit and illicit drugs *do*, which meant that 'leaving drugs alone' (a common phrase used by participants) was about more than leaving the potentiality of pleasure (rush-relief) alone, but leaving these life connections, of which, for some (seen most vehemently in Mya's account below), was something they would/could not contemplate or pursue.

For some participants, drug assemblages also played a role in enhancing life or in becoming some*body* else. Participants talked about how drugs enabled them to become friendlier, more energetic, tolerant and sociable to get out of themselves. But, like Deleuze (1978) and others (Biehl, 2010; Weinberg, 2013) have argued in relation to drugs, vital experimentations can turn into lethal experimentations, where these connections for living

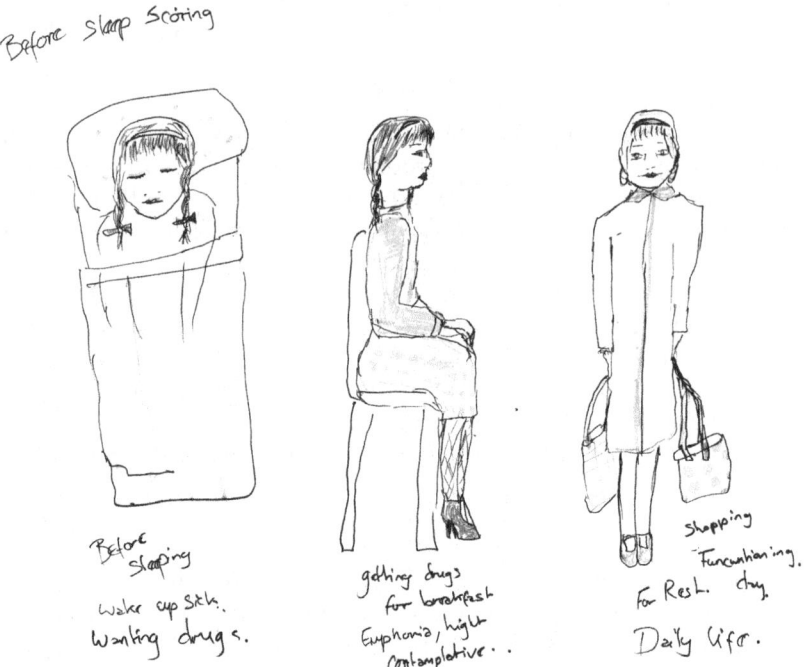

Figure 4.1 Sandra's body map depicts the role of drugs in her daily life.

get blocked. And participants often identified what Deleuze calls a 'turning point' between the two:

> That is also where all control is lost [de-stratification] and the system of abject dependence begins, dependence on the product, the hit, the fantasy productions, dependence on a dealer, etc. Two things must be distinguished, abstractly: the domain of vital experimentation, and the domain of deadly experimentation… It is the contrary of connection; it is organised *disconnection*.
>
> (1978: 153–4, my emphasis)

However, in my research, this threshold was nearly always conceived of in regard to dependency, often at the point of 'realising', which usually involved somebody else informing them that drugs (especially heroin) were 'needed' so not to be sick. I draw here on the extensive work of Peta Malins (2004; 2007; 2017), who also invokes Deleuze's more usual stance on bodies, rather than his more specific and uncharacteristically deterministic thinking on drugs. Deleuze not only seems to neglect the social dimensions in this 'turning point', but, in focussing on a process that is often seen as physical, has perhaps unwittingly slipped into a more classical account of the body. Participants talked about this change and identified a certain rigidification of affects (feeling, acting, thinking), but neither indicated a monolithic 'turning point' nor 'disconnection' that Deleuze and Guattari (1987) suggest. Vital connections did not exclusively turn into deadly connections. Although some connections were inevitably blocked, leaving participants feeling 'isolated' and 'trapped' (what Carlos felt as an 'invisible hold' and Jim as a 'curse'), as I see it, this is better conceived of as stratification, rather than de-stratification or disconnection (in his imagery of abject dependency). These processes are, of course, linked, but where the de-stratified body loses a connection to the assemblage – the derailed, 'vitrified' drugged body is alone and impermeable (Deleuze and Guattari, 1987: 150) – a rigidified, stratified body continues to connect, holding the assemblage to account and appreciating how desire flows to stratify (limit the potentials of) some bodies more than others. As Malins (2004) argues, the drug-using body is stratified as an 'addict' and 'junkie' in a way that prevents it from becoming-other. Stratification is caused when singularities are locked into systems, blocking the potential to transform into something else. Such processes are central to what Deleuze and Guattari (1983) call the 'control society' in which desire is 'machined' (cut or channelled) to produce individual subjects with restricted and often fixed identities and roles (e.g. 'drug user', 'addict', 'woman', 'British'). The examples of where bodies get stratified in their encounters with drug assemblages are countless, but here I focus on accounts of becoming blocked from becoming-other as 'a guest at a party', 'a boyfriend', 'an employee' and 'a patient'. As will become clear, it is in these *connections* with other bodies – of legislation, knowledge, imagery, etc. – rather than in de-stratification (where one connection [with-drug] takes over) that drugged bodies become blocked.

Therefore, in invoking a more characteristically Deleuzian approach, I take the desiring body– a machinic assemblage connected-up to numerous other bodies – as my starting point. In these assemblages, some connections are blocked, but this does not mean that others cannot open up. The way these bodies come together is a matter of encounter rather than inevitable course (from vital to deadly), of which, we too, as researchers and practitioners (to be continued in the following chapters), are part of, and thus should intervene to encourage as many good encounters and as few bad encounters as possible, whether this includes drugs or not.

Becoming 'normal'

People say, 'don't you ever want to come off?' I don't know. The thought of me getting up without taking something is totally… to me that's *normal*. If I haven't taken anything then *I'm not normal*. And for me to even, I can't contemplate not taking something, you know. I'm not a lost cause. I know what my problem is. It's other people that want me to stop. I don't want to stop. I don't want to. *Does that make sense to you?*

Mya, 52 years old, injects diamorphine

Mya has been injecting illicitly sought prescription diamorphine (pharmaceutical heroin) for over ten years and has recently started at a National Health Service specialist diamorphine clinic (as part of a randomised control trial), where they intended to reduce her consumption. However, this is not her intention, and she explains with a heavy heart how she is feeling this substantial pressure. She feels the clinic staff are failing to understand how 'drugs are part of her' and what constitutes her 'normal', and thus, her problem, as she sees it, is not the drugs themselves, but the people that want her to stop using them. In delivering this passage (above), Mya was visibly upset and it had taken her a long time to build up to this verbalisation. Her sentiment also resonated with several other participants (e.g. Lucy, Jim and Sandra) who were similarly distressed by the prospect of having to reduce or give up their prescribed or/and illicit drug consumption.

Following Foucault, the social sciences of medicine have for a long time critiqued the category of normal as socially constructed. That is, normality changes through time and space, and gets *performed* accordingly. In drug research, Nettleton and colleagues (2013) draw on Foucault, and his concept of governmentality, more specifically, to explore how 'recovering' heroin users employ a concept of normalisation in regaining certain bodily practices. Quoting Foucault (1977), 'normalisation' is seen as 'a crucial aspect of neoliberal societies, where individuals are encouraged through [decentralised] political projects to become normal: "the judges of normality are everywhere"' (Nettleton et al., 2013: 175).

However, Mya's narrative of becoming-normal seems to be doing something else. She highlights how she becomes normal *with* drugs in a way that without drugs she is 'not normal'. This highlights the *material* work involved in achieving this normal state. It is clear that being normal is something we *do* rather than being given or preordained, but, for Mya, this is enacted in an ontological way, as she connects with drugs, rather than only learnt socially. To *know* normality – 'to me that's normal' – and to *be* normal – 'if I haven't taken anything then I'm not normal' – are conflated, one of the same. This reflects Barad's (2007) agential realism, where what we *know* (epistemologically) and what *is* (ontologically) are part of the same process of becoming. It is in these entanglements of matter and meaning that Mya *becomes* normal. This 'becoming' starts to make more sense when we also think about the body as something we do, which, drawing on Mol and Law (2004), is involved in a constant task of *keeping oneself together*. This shifts attention from the pleasure assemblage (seen in the previous chapter) to assemblages for life and living.

'Keeping oneself together'

Participants talked about actively becoming ('holding together') *with drugs* – in ways that were life sustaining (becoming-normal) and life enhancing (becoming-other). Staying, for now, with the former, or what, for Vicki, in the account below, the dealers do not sometimes 'get', and in Mya's account (above), the service providers also did not, is that 'a lot of people' who use drugs live 'relatively normal lives' and hence, like Vicki, they 'want the up, the buzz' in order to go to work and 'keep things together'. Bodies are actively held together in practice (Mol, 2002; Mol and Law, 2004). Instead of drugs being seen as 'evil' objects of misuse, for Mya, they were part of this *vital* (life) project of keeping oneself together, which thoroughly blurs the distinctions between 'good' medicine (life sustaining/enhancing) and 'bad' drugs of abuse (life destroying) (Keane, 2002).

Following on from the idea that making the body actualise as *one* is a process of life, drugs, for some, were part of this boundary making.

> 'A' or 'a' (one) is always the index of a multiplicity: an event, a singularity, a life [...] A transcendent can always be invoked which falls outside the plane of immanence, or which attributes the plane to itself... nevertheless transcendence is always a product of immanence.
>
> (Deleuze, 1995a: 388)

For Mya, drugs were part of this individualisation process in extraordinarily overt ways. In her body map (Figure 4.2), she draws a picture of herself inside a cloud, with voices shouting at her, penetrating this protective barrier. She says, they are 'shouting at me', 'telling me what to do' and 'what's best for me'. But she was at pains to point out that the depicted cloud is not about representing a pleasurable or disassociated feeling – for experimenting with perception, in the ways that Deleuze and Guattari (1987) actually condone (Malins, 2017: 127) – but blocking out these intruding voices telling her how to live her life so that they 'can't get to me':

MYA: That makes it sound like the drug makes me feel like I'm in a cloud, it doesn't, cos I just feel *normal*, it just helps me to, to deal with things better, it helps me to get less stressful, does that make sense?

FD: Normal? (repeating her language).

MYA: Yeah.

FD: So, if you haven't had it, you feel more on edge?

MYA: I'm a complete nervous wreck. I'll be jumping everywhere, you know, if someone opens the window of a bus and I'm jumping.

For Mya, then, her drug use is not about pleasure, or removing pain, for that matter, but about something altogether more vital: keeping together in

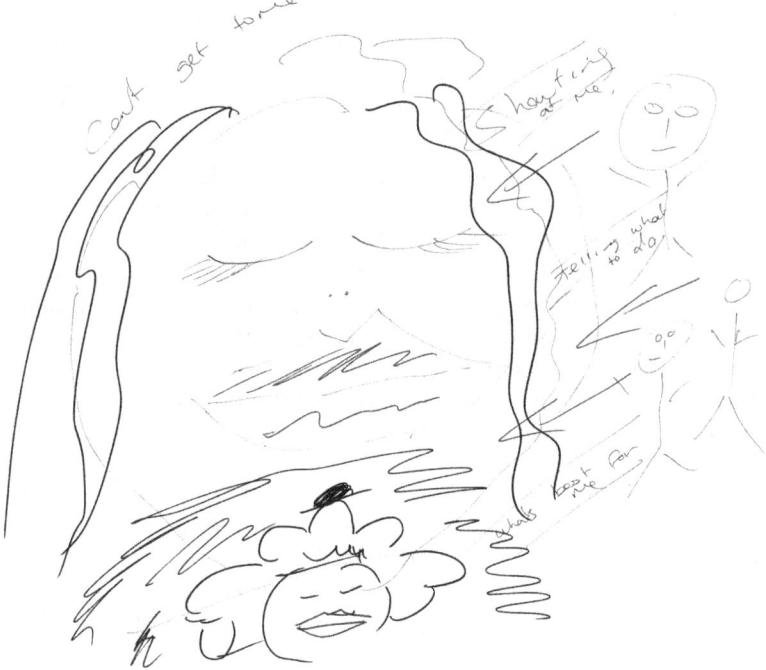

Figure 4.2 Mya's body map.

a stressful, invasive world, to 'deal with things better'. Drugs were intimately involved in trying to hold this 'active' body together.

> ...the active body has semi-permeable boundaries... inside and outside are not so stable. Metabolism, after all, is about eating, drinking and breathing; about defecating, urinating and sweating. For a metabolic body incorporation and excorporation are essential.
>
> (Mol and Law, 2004: 54)

A similar argument is made by Vitellone, citing Keane (2002):

> Heroin is not separate from but becomes central to the body, selfhood, and processes of *individualization*. Thus, according to Keane 'a drug is something external that becomes internalized, blurring the distinction between not only inside/outside but also self/other'.
>
> (Vitellone, 2003b: 166)

In Mya's drawing and account, drugs are intimately involved in the task of individuating, rather than say, de-stratifying – in making clear boundaries between her and the world in which the cloud acts like an extra layer of skin. Adding weight to this argument, Lucy similarly comments on how, without drugs, she does not feel herself, to the point that she said, 'I don't want to be in my own skin'. Simon also used similar language to note that, without heroin (even though he is prescribed methadone, an opiate substitute), he can feel 'disembodied' (see Figure A.2):

> Everything is all 'oh oh' [he makes sounds and body movements to show a fear of things getting too close] like that, everything is like right, like if you're trying to walk around the streets and it's just like you can't handle busy high streets and you know busy like tubes [underground transport system] and...

In these accounts, drugs are playing a key role in this boundary work, that is, in enacting the body as one. This resonates strongly with Haraway's concept of individualisation as 'a strategic defence problem' (1991b: 212). This is the idea that the individual body is not something we are born with, but something we strive towards. Haraway argues that 'bodies have become cyborgs', where 'the cyborg is text, machine, body, and metaphor' (ibid). Mya takes great care in making sure that I have understood this process of boundary-making, which is essential to the cyborg, and, on several occasions, checks back with me to confirm that she is making sense. She gives the impression that she has been explaining these feelings for years, but still does not feel fully understood. This is perhaps why she seemed so thrilled when she felt I had finally got a handle on the dynamic:

MYA: But the methadone makes me feel heavy, lethargic, with the diamorphine I can get on with *being normal, more better*, and not so sleepy, does that make sense? *It just helps me cope with everything.* You know what I mean, *everything.* Even...
FD: Like taking the edge off things?
MYA: That's it, the edge off things, you've got it! I've never thought of that before, that's a good way of putting it.
FD: No cos I was thinking about what you were saying about how you can feel anxious and stuff, and I can imagine it just... [cut off]
MYA: You're right, you've done it in a nut shell there. Cos people have asked me that before and I haven't been able to answer. That is a good answer. It takes the edge of things. Yeah.

At the end of the interview, and long past this initial reference, Mya shows appreciation of this phrase once more, as an expression which she feels could help in her bid to be better understood:

FD: Anyway, I'll end the interview there.
MYA: Was that alright?

FD: Yeah, perfect. Is there anything else that you think is important that I've missed out?

MYA: No not at all. I think you've just helped me there by saying it takes the edge off things, I've been trying to put that into words for a long time, I didn't know how to say it...

Although these accounts of holding together are, of course, linked to withdrawal symptoms as a particular arrangement of bodily connections that need continually re-aligning, when I ask about this, it is evident that it is also about something more. In trying to get at why Mya feels she needs diamorphine rather than methadone (which would be the more usual opiate prescribed in heroin treatment), she talks about it being 'cleaner', 'purer', 'less groggy'. And even though I prompted her on the potential enjoyment of diamorphine over methadone, she links 'the buzz' to being able to get on with 'normal things', which contributes to her normality, saying 'I can act more normal with the heroin' [diamorphine]:

MYA: Definitely, it's less groggy.

FD: And does it give you a slight buzz also?

MYA: Sometimes it does yeah. Like I can get on with my housework better and things like that, day to day things, I can act more *normal* with the heroin. With just the methadone, things just *slip*.

With an interesting use of the term, Mya says that with methadone 'things just slip'. There is a sense in which diamorphine is holding her together, in a way that without it she would 'slip'. This perhaps highlights again the slipperiness of connections that are only ever partial (Haraway, 1991a: 181). Rather than becoming too porous, with methadone she becomes too shut off or 'groggy', and again her body becomes unable to do things. This is why she is so insistent that diamorphine stays put in her life: 'I'm not going to lie, even if I don't get it [prescribed], I'm still going to use the diamorphine'. Or, in Haraway's words, she 'would rather be a cyborg than a goddess' (1991a: 181) – she would rather endure the political and potentially criminal consequences of requiring this external substance than pretend to live apart from/ above the material world.

Mya's account of drug use as keeping oneself together thoroughly disrupts a separation of the object from the subject, as well as several other problematic binaries that underpin contemporary ideas of drug use and the body, including drug/medicine, inner/outer, self/other and, of course, what constitutes what is considered normal and pathological. Instead, she does not want to give diamorphine up as her body is connected with it in a way that holds her together (as one) in becoming 'normal'. Consequently, the threat of having these drugs stopped pose a very real, ontological risk to their embodied corporeality, which demands to be taken seriously.

Pushing further on this idea of the body as something we do, then health too is also something we do. And, as such, for many participants, drugs were not so much about pleasure (rush-relief) or becoming normal but becoming healthier. This starts to make more sense when we think about health through Deleuze's concept of a 'power of acting' (Duff, 2014a).

Doing 'health'

Contrary to dominant discourses, some participants positioned their drug use in terms of sustaining life or 'becoming' in healthier ways. This resonates with Duff's (2014a) reorientation of health as a matter of life, where attention is shifted from 'the body' to a Deleuzian ethics of affect (ethico-aesthetics), which potentialises the body to act as its ability to affect and be affected:

> Health [...] may be understood to involve those forms of bodily activity that extend a body's range of action – construed as the array of bodies, entities, things and processes that such a body may affect and/or be affected by – along with the variety of human and nonhuman, organic and material relations that subtend this activity.
>
> (Duff, 2014a: 75)

Within this broader frame of affect, we can start to take more seriously participant's accounts of using drugs for health and well-being, seen here, to improve symptoms of physical illness and emotional trauma and stress. Where this could be dismissed as a neoliberal desire to stratify, to fit into socially sanctioned roles and identities, I wish to argue that it is also about something more creative. By rethinking how drug use is positioned as health destroying, this could reduce some of the negative effects in how drugs get known and done, and the consequences (such as prison sentences). Widening our understanding of drugs beyond such a formulation allows for their multiplicitous enactments (the differences in how drugs get done and experienced) and thereby reduces some of the harms produced in its narrow composition.

Sandra, introduced above was forty-eight years old and had been injecting heroin on and off since she was twenty-two. She explains that she has health problems, and has 'maintained' her current heroin use of injecting once to twice a day to help ease these issues:

SANDRA: I've just managed to maintain it. What happened is, me and Gwen [have] both got the same thing, we've got COPD [chronic obstructive pulmonary disease] so we can't breathe without gear [heroin], it suppresses your breathing which really helps. We can't breathe without the gear. And also, I've got a degenerative back problem so I can't walk without it. I could not walk, I couldn't walk at all.

FD: Did they put you on methadone in jail?

SANDRA: Yeah. I was only on 9 ml, so they kept me under the 10 so I wouldn't withdraw. But then everything started going wrong. I could hardly walk. I take heroin and I can walk. I can't walk. And there's not going to give me a substitute, because I'm a drug user (she starts crying). I can't go to the GP [General Practitioner] because she'll tell the probation and then they'll lock me up for using drugs.

Up until this point, Sandra was answering the questions confidently and was very talkative, telling me about her prison sentence and time 'serving up' (drug dealing), but suddenly with the mention of how much heroin was helping her and the thought of not getting a substitute, she started to cry.

Sandra was on licence for drug-dealing charges, she knows that if her probation worker finds out she is using, she would be found in breach of her conditions of release and could be sent back to prison. Tangentially, Sandra was also in critical need of hospital treatment for an abscess, but too afraid to attend due to the real fear that she would not be given any substitute mediation or would be ousted as 'a drug user'. Interestingly, it is her identity – '*I am* a drug user' – rather than say her practices of drug use that she is suggesting prevents these other ways of being, for example, a patient who is able to get the care she requires. Sandra is left in an impossible situation in which she feels unable to seek professional help. For now at least, she is going to continue using illicit heroin to walk and feel more able to do things. However, her abscesses may not improve without medical care, and hence her tears and desperation. This predicament exemplifies how harms can manifest through such an identity.

Gwen (mentioned in Sandra's account), who is a close friend of Sandra, similarly explains how heroin is helping her:

> at the moment I'm happy to carry on because I'm not very well anyway and it helps me, *it helps me get through the day*. I can admit that I actually like doing it, because I'm having a miserable life with my illnesses. I've got Crohn's disease and the thing about Crohn's is that you have constant diarrhoea and pain. Heroin and morphine constipates you so it stops the diarrhoea so I'm actually using it medicinally as well. They say that if we could prescribe you morphine for your condition we would but we're not allowed to.

Heroin helps Gwen 'get through the day' both medicinally for her chronic health conditions and in offering enjoyment. So, for Gwen, just because she uses drugs for medicinal and health sustaining reasons does not mean that it is not pleasurable – the two are by no means mutually exclusive. Both

Sandra and Gwen explain that their health conditions are chronic and will eventually become terminal.

> I've got COPD, so I probably won't live longer than 5–6 years, because it's irreversible, your lungs are fucked. So basically, I'm happy to stay as I am for the minute [injecting heroin], I'm not going to ruin myself any further [pause]. As long as I don't bother anyone and I can manage my bills.
>
> (Gwen)

They both feel that they want to continue using heroin to manage these conditions. Furthermore, the process of injecting, which can often be overlooked as a route of administration, was firmly embedded in this 'becoming'. In highlighting her aversion to drug services and their harm reduction interests, Sandra exclaims:

> They just tell you to smoke it and I said no I can't smoke it, I haven't got time to smoke it, I'm working, how can I have time to smoke it, what do I take it to work, are you crazy! Are you crazy! This will happen, that will happen and all that they do is they tell you loads of things that will happen [the risks associated with injecting] but they don't tell you what will happen with the foil, you can get aluminium build up, you can get loads of crap.

The injecting assemblage (syringe, cooker, water, citric, alcohol wipes, venous system) cannot be detached from those other bodies (e.g. substance) in becoming-healthier (at least less pained) as a heightened capacity to act or literately moved 'through the day' in being able to walk. Smoking, in fact, as Sandra sees it, will only get in the way of such movement as a more time-consuming route of administration.[1] She is extremely frustrated with workers who fail to understand this as if it is only the ingestion of the substance (by any means) that matters and not what it enables her to do.

With the same distain and mistrust as Sandra treats smoking, methadone was also not an option:

FD: So, you wouldn't go back to methadone then?

SANDRA: Are you crazy! It doesn't function, it takes three days to get in your body so when you're sick, it doesn't do anything and it's hard to keep down so the crisis is over by the time it works, well you think it is...

It was through injecting that both Sandra and Gwen felt they could incorporate heroin into their bodies in the safest, quickest and most enjoyable way.

In a comparable way to how heroin acted 'medicinally' for Gwen and Sandra's physical health conditions (Crohn's, COPD, back pain), for other participants, drugs acted as an emotional crutch and a creative way of coping with difficult life circumstances.

> It did help actually did the crack, during that time when I was recovering from the break up. I mean, you think, sometimes, I know self-medicating is not the answer, but it did actually help me at the time–and I'll stand by that [...] – to get through [pause] each day, you know, *instead of wanting to die,* you know, and *not carry on.*
>
> (Vicki)

Vicki explains how crack helped her 'to get through' a difficult period in her life. In this instance, it helped her to hold together, and 'carry on', where to stop could have been fatal. Demonstrating the ontological significance of Mol and Law's (2004) sentiment from the epigraph, it kept her together and, in this, alive. In connecting with other bodies (she explicitly names crack, but also her children: 'I mean the kids always got me through those times'), she was able to stay together and get on with things (her agency comes from this coming together of bodies). 'I just got into a routine with crack, keeping busy with it, you know'. Unlike heroin, which brought Vicki 'in on herself' (which, in contrast to Simon and Lucy [above], made the distinction between the self and other too stark), crack kept her busy, offered her a routine and, with this, kept her engaged with the world, so she could get through the break-up and take care of her children.

With a similar recourse to self-medication, Mason identifies his heroin use as a way of coping with a childhood trauma and ongoing post-traumatic stress. In this, he positions his use of heroin as a positive change in his life. Contrary again to dominant discourses, he considers heroin, which is widely considered one of the most harmful drugs (in Class A under the Misuse of Drugs Act 1971), to be better for him than his previous use of ketamine (which is in Class B) and other so-called 'softer' or 'recreational' drugs (e.g. marihuana, ecstasy). Mason explains how his encounters with drugs are different from other people. The ways his body (and the history it has) assembles will produce different affects or ways of feeling, thinking and acting. Again, as has been reiterated throughout the book, it is not the drug that is intrinsically good/bad, but how it comes together and connects-up with other bodies in the drug-using assemblage (Duff, 2014a; Keane, 2002; Malins, 2004). 'Instead of a moral distinction between substances as good or evil, healthy or unhealthy, the question would be one of either good or bad encounters [...]. The challenge is to increase the good encounters and limit the bad, just as we do in other relationships' (Keane, 2002: 35).

As participants imaginatively and inventively, often against states of oppression and exploitation, seek to increase good encounters and limit the bad, it is too simplistic to understand this dynamic in terms of 'self-medication'. Although, perhaps one of the least problematic models of addiction, that is, it is less judgemental/moralising than the 'choice model' and less pathologising than the 'disease model' (Lewis, 2012), it still has significant issues. First it fails to take seriously the vast array of life-affirming reasons why people use drugs. But more problematically, it relies on the self as distinct from the non-human other ('medication'). By taking the body and health as something we do, this theorem is substantially weakened. Following Duff's reading of Deleuze, health is as much external as internal, cultural as natural and made up of both subjects and objects:

> Human life (the embodied subject) is involuted. 'Implicated' in this process of folding by which an 'inside' (or interiority) like mind, consciousness or subjectivity is produced in a 'differential synthesis' of an always present, always folded 'outside' that includes the folds of habit, practice, sense data, food, water, other bodies, ideas, technologies.
>
> (Deleuze, 1994: 70–4, cited in Duff, 2014a: xii)

There is no outside and inside that is not made and therefore we cannot start from the premise of subjects or bodies as separate from objects or medicine. The fact that everyone is in a constant state of self-medication, incorporating and excorporating, in becoming more or less active (affected and affecting), renders the concept moot. Such a concept of human life can also lead to a radical de-pathologisation of drug use without disposing of the fact that not all encounters are good.

Where professionals are unwilling or unable to facilitate good drug encounters in line with a rigid legal and moral framework based on specific drugs as bad, navigating these encounters are largely left up to users themselves. For Mason, like other participants, heroin, which is arguably the drug most vilified in most societies, produces benefits and is regularly part of good encounters. I will quote a large excerpt from our conversation as this gives a better sense of his position.

FD: Would you say that your drug use has changed over the years... has it got heavier or slowed down a bit or...?

MASON: It's got a hell of a lot better, because I used to do loads, thinking about it, and I'm not doing any of that anymore. I used to do 50 grams a week of ketamine, so [pause] very, very rough times they were, but great times because I was off my face all the time, excellent.

FD: So now you don't use ketamine at all?

MASON: Don't touch it. Don't touch marihuana, ecstasy, speed, nothing like that

FD: So, you almost feel like it's better just on the brown [heroin]?

MASON: Yeah, it's more chilled out. There's just, I've done all that before, you get bored of it.

FD: And what would you say, it's a weird question, but what would you say your main reasons for using drugs are now?

MASON: Blocking, and enjoyment, and relaxation.

FD: And do you feel like it's something that you're in control of or do you feel like the drugs are in control of you? Do you know what I mean?

MASON: Well, it's a bit of both, well obviously if I don't have it I'm sick so there's that element of control, I'm always going to need it because of that, but, yeah, the thing is, *I'm more dependent on it because of the blocking, that's why I really do it*, I haven't done anything else that really works as well, and sometimes [the prescribed medicine] makes it worse. It [the heroin] *makes it a hell of a lot better,* you know, the stress and anxieties so, so yeah, *so in that sense it controls me because it's my medication.*

Mason describes his positive encounters with heroin, which only make sense and materialise as such in relation to his past trauma, ongoing anxieties and lack of any better medication, making him feel 'a hell of a lot better'. He specifically highlights that this is about more than relieving withdrawal symptoms:

> That's not a result of the withdrawal [he points to the image of him before using drugs on his body map, see Figure A.3]. I've been diagnosed with bipolar and PTSD [Post-Traumatic Stress Disorder] as well. And I'm not on medication. Well, I was given some medication, but I didn't like it very much because of the way it made me feel. It made me feel drowsy, in a really lethargic kind of way. Whereas *I can function on this much better, and it actually makes it a hell of a lot better, it's incredible.*

Using Duff's (2014a) broader notion of health, we can start to think about the different roles that drugs play and how public health, to remain relevant, needs to respond to and allow for these differences. Instead of heroin being intrinsically bad, in these specific encounters, for Mason, it is felt as medicine-like, and he says: 'at the end of the day, if I want to medicate myself, I'll medicate myself'. So, for Mason, like Mya, Gwen, Sandra and others, heroin was a substance that could enact positive effects and was therefore not something they wished to give up. In this sense (and in a similar way to Gwen and Sandra), Mason described drug services as having nothing to offer him. Consequently, he did not use them, even to the point that he served a prison sentence instead of a Drug Rehabilitation Requirement[2] (which would have required him to evidence a willingness to stop using): 'basically my argument was that I'm going to carry on using and at the end of the day you may as well send me to jail'.

During another point of the interview with Vicki, she highlighted the role drugs played in her work life: 'It's more energy with me I think, cos I like to work, I hate, I psychologically hate not working, y'know'. As stated in her quote at the beginning of the chapter, this is what Vicki says dealers do not understand in typecasting all heroin users as wanting the same thing: 'dealers always make the mistake in thinking that heroin users want one thing and that's to be out of it'. But, she explains, 'not everyone is like that, a lot of people want the up, buzz, as well, lots of people go to work, working, living relatively normal lives, y'know, they have things to keep together'. Heroin is used for more than escaping the world ('to be out of it'), but also engaging with it, and used in ways to harness agency, 'to keep together', and for living 'relatively normal lives'.

As well as the substance, the practice of injecting itself was crucial to the drug encounter as a life-sustaining/normalising practice. Injecting was experienced to have a longer period of influence: 'The other thing about fixing is that it lasts twelve hours, if you smoke, you're sick after six to eight hours, you've got to do it more frequently' (Gwen). Sandra also found injecting to be faster and easier than other routes, which made it more amenable for working and living 'normally'. Tom sums this sentiment up when he says: 'I mean really it's only like ten minutes out of the day that you don't lead a normal life'. It was in this specific connection of the genetic body (vein, blood, nervous system) with the substance and injecting equipment (syringe, etc.) that more controllable affects were produced. This not only questions intravenous drug use as the most destructive form of drug administration, but also challenges popular images, seen especially in social realist films, of sequential pharmacokinetic trajectories. Writing in response to this genre that was prevalent in the 1990s, including films such as Pure, Vitellone, through Keane, argues:

> *Pure* mirrors the sequential logic of the medical model of addiction involving 'predictable stages' (Keane, 2002: 39) and 'a notion of temporal development' (Keane, 2002: 40), a model which Keane points out is inscribed on the body itself. (2004: 144)

Citing Keane, for Vitellone, this 'reinforce[s] the idea that drug dependence is a different order of things from normal attachment to daily routines and habits, and normal preoccupation with certain activities' (2002: 55, cited in Vitellone, 2004: 145). In contrast to these representations, participants' accounts in my study considered heroin as central, even essential to these 'normal attachments'.

There is a mode of intra-corporeality or intra-subjectivity to injecting, which meant it also became part of human relationships and sharing to be 'on the same level' together. Gwen tells me:

> Me and [Sandra] try and keep ourselves to ourselves, but she was in prison for two years and during that time I stopped fixing. And then she

came out and I started again. It's not her fault at all I asked her to do it. *Especially where we're sharing*, once you've cut a bag in half there's not much to go round. So, I said I might as well have a hit, it lasts 12 hours whereas I would be me needing it again 8 hours down the line and she being alright for 12 hours. So it's kind of like, *we're on the same level* so we tend to do that.

Being 'on the same level' was an important aspect to Gwen's using with Sandra. Where current public health technologies and knowledge try to individualise subjects, this helps reinvigorate a dividual (collectivist) account where using is a shared experience (Fraser, 2013).

In this section, I have tried to highlight the many ways that drugs were getting done, where they were not being used explicitly or exclusively for pleasure, but for something more mundane, that is, for living and sustaining normal lives, including health, coping, working and even human relationships. In considering bodies as something we do rather than have, I have shown some of the ways drugs are felt to produce and sustain life. In these accounts, there is a disruption of the binaries that often organise drug use as illicit/licit, drug/medicine, and human life as inner/outer, self/other, and thus what is considered normal/pathological. But as well as bodies connecting with drugs in a way to sustain life, for others, drugs played an active role in becoming-other, in opening up new and exciting connections beyond the tedium of the everyday, and in this sense, they were also felt to be life enhancing.

Becoming-other

How it makes you feel? My mates say, when I haven't had nothing I'm quiet, and then as soon as I've had something *I'm completely changed*. My mood's like up, and I'm taking the piss and everything like that, complete, like you can spot it, you can, *the complete change is like yeah, totally different*.

Dimitri, 41 years old, injects heroin

For some participants, the positive effects of the drug assemblage were felt more as a change in subjectivity (in becoming-other) than a stabilising of subjectivity (in becoming-normal or healthy). However, there is a fine line between the two as both are underpinned by an ontology of process, that is, 'stabilising' should not be confused with anything static. Even so, some participants saw their drug use more in terms of experimenting with life, in an enhancing way, in becoming somebody else.

Becoming-other is established via 'diversity, multiplicity [and] the destruction of identity' (Deleuze, 1995b: 44); it presupposes breaking out

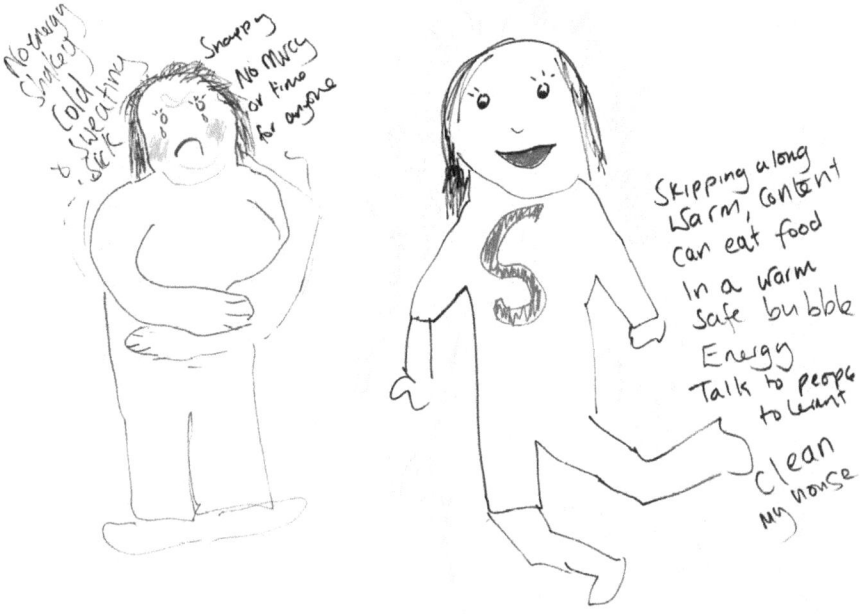

Figure 4.3 Meg's body map. She emphasises a change in self from without drugs to with them.

of our old outlived habits and attitudes so as to creatively 'bring into being that which does not exist' (Deleuze, 1994: 147).

(Semetsky, 2011: 139)

This becoming-other is also slightly different from the immediate pleasurable effects of 'the hit'. As I said, this is more about desire than pleasure, where desire brings us into connection with others in new ways. In this sense, like Malins (2017) recently argued, pleasure is only one aspect of desire, a materialisation of desire which is in fact a closing down of desire. Participants described becoming a different kind of self or de-stratification. Dimitri, in the quote above, accounts for his drug use in a way that allowed him to become some*body* else – he describes a 'complete change'. He feels more energised, jovial and friendly, highlighting the de-stratifying potential of drugs to break down fixed identities and roles. Instead of addiction or dependency, indeed he is on an opiate substitute that should prevent withdrawal symptoms, and he accounts for his use in terms of countering the tedium of the everyday:

A lot of it is boredom, a lot of it is boredom, I go to a place called T [a community day centre] in [north London] and I've got a key worker

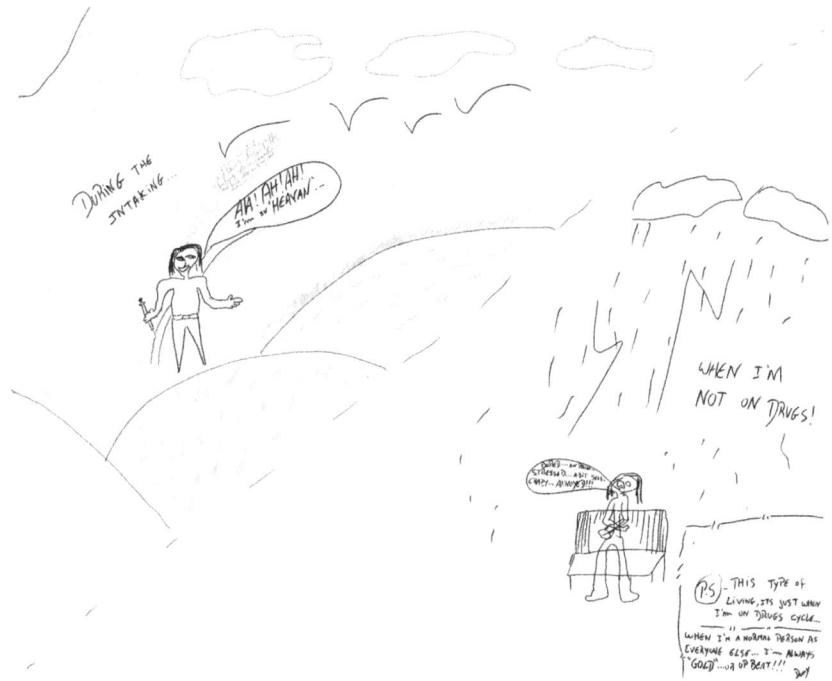

Figure 4.4 Carlos's body map. He depicts a change in relation to the world from being without to being with drugs. The speech bubble on the right says: 'bored, in pain, stressed, a bit self-crazy, annoyed'. And the left one says: 'I'm ecstatic, happy, and would love to always be feeling as disconnected and friendly as I am now'.

there and I talk to him and I say 'look, I cannot sit in this place just normal, when I sit in this place I'm just bored', and I just wanna use. And then, once I've had something, I can sit there.

For Dimitri, drugs are not about becoming-normal, in fact, he explicitly does not wish to be 'normal', but neither are they explicitly about pleasure. Instead, they allowed him to become in a way that made these mundane daily encounters more bearable. Similar changes were described by Meg and Carlos. Their body maps above (Figure 4.3 and 4.4) clearly depict this becoming-other, for Meg, from misery to feeling like superwoman, and for Carlos, from being enveloped by rain clouds to sunshine. Whilst these changes in subjectivity are undoubtedly linked to withdrawal symptoms, it is again about more than this. For Meg, her transformation was evidently into something more than herself, that is, more than feeling better or normal. She explained to me how her encounters with drugs (usually injecting heroin and smoking crack) and the world (with people and things [e.g. her house]) made her feel like 'superwoman': more energised, active (in that she felt more motivated to clean her house), friendly ('can talk to people') and 'tolerant'.

For Carlos, there was a similar transformative quality in his interactions with drugs, in which he talks about changing from a 'shy person' to a 'mini fly', who could take on a 'big bee':

> Because, for example, drugs have this image of being 'bad boy' sort of thing you know, so I start taking a bit more and *people started to look at me a bit differently*, cos I was a *shy person* then, and then when I start taking coke *I was more active more...* Sometimes I would even take on guys two or three times my size, two or three of them, and people think wow, look at that *mini fly* taking on that big bee, because I was just so out of my mind on, *it would give me balls*.

From being somebody who was shy, he became more active, confident and seemingly powerful, both physically and socially. The image of the 'bad boy' played an important part in this change. His self-perception was intricately linked with the perception of others – such external and internal forces are not divorced, but intimately intra-related. By connecting-up with this image of the 'bad boy', Carlos became something else – a mini fly. His confidence grew, people started to look at him differently and he could fight guys two or three times his size. Within this particular drug assemblage, the image proved to be just as important as the cocaine ingested.

This powerful drugged body, which had learnt to be affected and affect through the drug assemblage, reached its pinnacle at a festival, described as 'paradise', amongst an array of bodies, images, discourse and non-human matter – a 'gorgeous' girl, dealing drugs, earning lots of money, and sniffing and injecting cocaine:

> And then one day I met a girl and she was gorgeous, she was very funny, she was very friendly, and she used to sniff a lot. So I booked two tickets, we went to [an island] – it was a big, big rave and I took 15 grams of coke and then one guy was looking for me, I called him and he brought a bit more and I was there a few hours and I was by the speakers and groups were coming over, 5–10 guys, then 5–10 guys then [pause to symbolise the excitement and movement] you know in 5–10 minutes, you do a grand, just like that. I'd give to my girl, she'd go out, come back, and then another 5 minutes, £500 to a grand [thousand pounds], 'poof'. In a few hours, I'd done 4–5 grand. And then everyone was coming over 'oh [Carlos], this is good, have a line with me', and then after a while it was snowballing (injecting), and then we spent a week, it was paradise.

Other participants similarly accounted for a sense of excitement in this newly found drug world (connecting to the image and substance). Jim talks about the missed lifestyle that got him back into using drugs after a period of abstinence: 'But you do get those sorts of things, buzzes, and I missed all that life, and it did excite me, like getting back into crime and that, more than the drugs'. And Mya accounted for the way drugs enabled a more exciting lifestyle in terms of the 'fast lane'. But she is very clear that where there were openings (becoming-other) in the form of posh hotels, owning her own car, having disposable income, there were also closings – 'the gutter' and eventually prison.

> It's the fast lane, isn't it. You know what I mean, I had a lot of working girls who were my friends, I was going from one hotel to the next, I've been in the Ritz, I've been in the Dorchester, I've been in the gutter, you know, it's the fast world.

For both Carlos and Mya, in Deleuze's (1978) terms, vital connections started becoming lethal connections. But there was no 'turning point' in the way Deleuze describes.

> How do we account for a 'turning point' in drugs, how do we determine at what moment this turning point occurs? [...] The drug use creates active lines of flight. But these lines roll up, start to turn into black holes, with each drug user in a hole, as a group or individually, like a periwinkle. Dug in instead of spaced out....
>
> (Deleuze, 1978: 253)

For Mya, there were lines of flight alongside blockages, and rather than a 'turning' from one to the other, there were multiple connections, some good and some bad. Mya had not ended her illicit drug use because it had become deadly but had just started using different drugs (licit diamorphine and methadone) and in a different way (through an injecting clinic), which meant they became less dangerous (no risk of imprisonment) although more inconvenient (she has to travel a long way). They have become about sustaining this 'normal' state rather than either enhancing life (vital experimentation) or destroying it (lethal experimentation): 'I don't look funny! I need it just to function normally you know'. But where drugs were still working for Mya, for keeping together and living normally, for others they were not.

For Carlos, this turning point could at first seem more applicable, with the 'island rave' marking this change in direction. Before the party, he says he was dealing low quantities and only consuming small amounts – 'maybe I would take one tiny line, tiny line, once every couple of months, at big, big parties'. But then, immediately following the island party, he explains how his using started to spiral:

> And then we got back [home], she went back to her boyfriend, and that's when I realised what I was getting myself into. But by then I was loving that feeling, and then I started getting more and more and more, my friends started noticing, they started moving away.

However, where Carlos's account of paradise soon turned into something altogether bleaker, what is interesting, and a limitation to Deleuze's (1978) commentary on the topic, is that pleasure did not go away, and hence these vital and deadly lines of flight, like in Mya's account, rather than turning from one to the other, could coexist. Therefore, I turn now to these blocked 'becomings', but in a way that does not consign drug-using bodies to the dark holes of periwinkles.

Becoming-blocked: 'you don't grow'

> Within each drug assemblage, the body connects up not only to the drug (its texture, its smell, its taste, its appearance, its speed) but also to other bodies and machines–people, substances, knowledges, institutions – any of which may redirect or *block* its flows of desire.
>
> Peta Malins, 2004: 89, my emphasis

Jon's body map (Figure 4.5) vividly highlights some of the ways that participants were blocked from becoming-other. For Jon, this is namely felt in relation to having 'no girlfriend', 'no friends', 'no family' and being 'smelly, unwashed, hungry and homeless'. Deleuze's ontology of becoming is useful here for thinking about the ways that some drug connections can take over other ways of being. It is important to note that Deleuze is just as interested in the points where lines of flight converge and become blocked as he is in the points of flight. This is where, in his critical address to Michel Foucault, power is produced (Deleuze, 1977). As already mentioned, Deleuze has written specifically on these issues in relation to the drugged body in terms of blocked flows of desire and vital connections becoming lethal connections. Resonating with this, 'you don't grow' was a statement made by Silvie in relation to how she feels her drug use has made her unaffected by the ebbs and flows of ordinary life. It has prevented her moving and feeling through life, or in Deleuze's language, has blocked her flows of desire, in a way that makes her feel like time has stood still:

> Look at me like now, I've wasted all these years, so, before buying, you just think, in this time, you've done nothing, you've wasted all

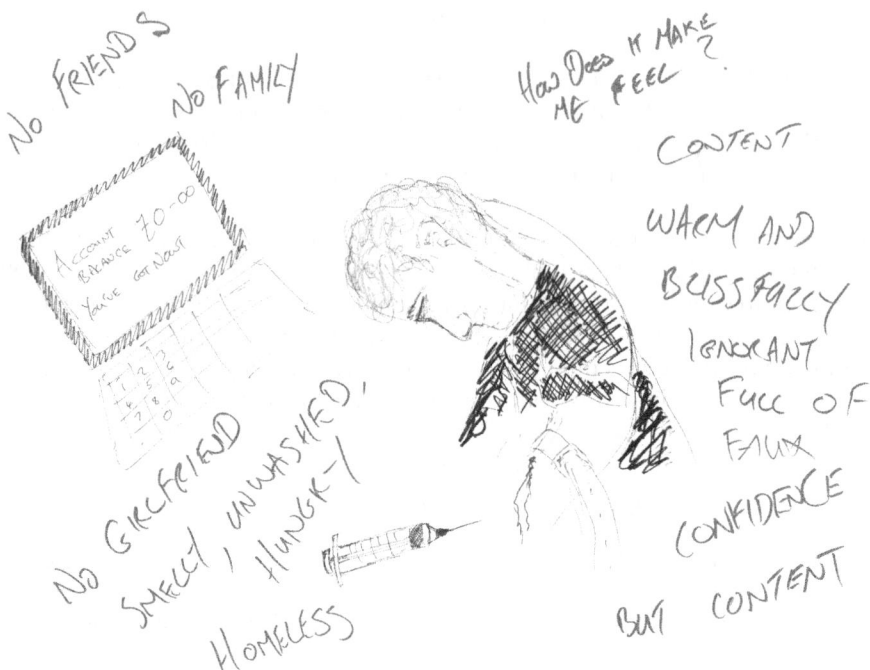

Figure 4.5 Jon's body map.

days by just buying something, going home, and you don't do any-thing, it's always tomorrow, tomorrow, tomorrow. Your life doesn't change, you stay, emotionally, like when you started using. You don't change, you stay like that, you don't grow emotionally, you stay the same, you don't go through, you don't cry, you don't get upset, you don't care about people, relationships, that's what I mean, you don't grow.

However, following Malins (2004), instead of using Deleuze's specific and uncharacteristically pessimistic account on drugged bodies, which consid-ers these blockages as matters of disconnection, I turn to his more general philosophical work on the assemblage and stratification (1994; and with Guattari, 1983; 1987), in arguing that, conversely, these blockages are a mat-ter of connection. That is, these negative affects get produced in connection with other bodies (human, material, imagined and discursive). I will first consider how this could rethink dependency or addiction and then go on to illustrate some more specific ways drug assemblages enact blockages as a guest at a party, a boyfriend, an employee and a patient.

In Deleuze's writing on the 'drugged body' in *Two Questions on Drugs* and with Guattari in *A Thousand Plateaus* he can be seen to be creating the very image of certainty he otherwise fought against:

> Instead of making a body without organs sufficiently rich or full for the passage of intensities, drug addicts erect a vitrified or emptied body, or a cancerous one: the causal line, creative line, or line of flight immediately turns into a line of death and abolition.
>
> (1987: 285)

The drugged body is seen to be a 'sucked dry' 'body-without-organs' (BWO) that is deplete of organisation, what Deleuze (cited at the beginning) alludes to in its disconnection: 'The *drugged body*... [is] a dreary parade of sucked-dry, catatonicized, vitrified, sewn-up bodies... Emptied bodies instead of full ones... What happened? Were you cautious enough?... Many have been defeated in this battle' (Deleuze and Guattari, 1987: 150).

But as I have already shown, participants' accounts challenge any unilinear idea of the turning point, which strangely resembles something more akin to the body-we-have or biological body. In many ways, Deleuze's commentary on drugged bodies slips into a transcendental logic, away from immanence. Indeed, here, I continue this argument in considering how participants' experiences of physical dependency were a product of bad connections (in the encounter), beyond any locked-in connection ('a line of death'). For example, even in Dimitri's near-fatal encounter with drugs, it is in a connection with the legal system that makes the people he was with question whether to ring for an ambulance. It is in these connections that a lethal line was brought about.

> The first time I injected, I nearly killed myself. I overdosed, and the house that I was in, they just left me. If it had been a little bit more, I would have like killed myself. I was out cold. Then, like hours later, I come around and we had an argument about whether you ring the ambulance cos I could have died and all that.

So, rather than disconnection, I see these harms, including addiction, as a matter of encounter, and, crucially, encountering bodies with 'stratifying' tendencies.

> Strata are Layers, Belts. They consist of giving form to matters, or imprisoning intensities or locking singularities into systems of resonance and redundancy, of producing upon the body of the earth molecules large and small and organising them into molar aggregates.
>
> (Deleuze and Guattari, 1987: 40)

That is, in connecting-up with media images, certain policies, biomedical knowledges, as well the substance and genetic material, and other bodies, including human and non-human, the drug-using body gets stratified as an addict, which limits other ways of 'becoming'. In overdosing, Dimitri was connected to the stratifying image of the addict or junkie, along with juris-dictional bodies, which contributed to the fact that those around him failed to call an ambulance fearing judgement and arrest.

In another example, Jim starts an account of his drug use, in a way similar to perhaps many 'addicts' (and in line with Deleuze's abject BWO), in terms of a loss of control ('cursed with it'). All his interests have become inconse-quential amounting to that one connection:

> Because by that time I knew that heroin had *got me,* cocaine *got me,* it wouldn't matter what I got in the world, nothing mattered. I was always into cars, motorbikes, but it wouldn't have mattered if somebody gave me a formula one car, it would have just been a car, as soon as I saw it I would have just thought cor that's worth about 40,000 bags of gear, do you know, everything was calculated that way.

But interestingly, it quickly becomes obvious that this is not a case of 'disor-ganisation' (as Deleuze would suggest), but an effect of the assemblage – a connection between not only drugs and the genetic body, but other bodies:

> …it's weird, because you almost think your cursed with it because I know if I gave it up tomorrow for the next 6 months I would be getting offered it every day, people would be saying 'you wanna try this'.

In this sense, dealers were also very much involved in this loss of control.

Following on from the previous chapter, this develops an understanding of addiction as a matter of shared control that is a folding of inner and outer worlds in acquiring habits and practices beyond the self. In elaborat-ing on his feeling of being 'cursed', it is the dealers that Jim cites in making his using so persistent rather than any single connection to the substance itself. For many participants, owning a mobile phone (often a prerequisite for buying drugs) also meant a constant onslaught of text messages adver-tising drugs which meant, even if they did not want to buy anything that day, it was made very hard to escape. Gwen's mobile phone goes off in the interview:

GWEN: 'J', see that's a dealer, 'J's on with 10/10', they send these to your phone man, it's ridiculous.
FD: With ten out of ten?
GWEN: Yeah, meaning they've got good stuff. I hate it when they do that, I delete it. I don't want that sort of stuff on my phone. I'll just delete it. I know who that is, that's one of the people that I've been going to.

FD: That's what other people have said, they get texts all the time.

GWEN: Advertising. If you don't want to use and somebody sends you that, especially if you've got no money, you start thinking where can I get some.

Crystal similarly comments on this situation, which makes it difficult not to use for the day:

> I like to think I'm in control most of the time, but all it can take is a text from a dealer or something like that to just trigger and then I think oh, fuck it, I'm going to go and get something.

This invokes a topological approach to space, that is, what counts is not metric distance but how closely entities are connected in an assemblage. 'Space, from this perspective, becomes folded or crumpled, almost like a handkerchief, whose ends, if laid out flat on a table, are far from each other but end up close together when scrunched' (Müller, 2015: 35). Perhaps, unsurprisingly then, mobile phones became a central part of some body maps (like Silvie's [Figure 4.6], see also Lucy's, Chapter 3), where these 'becomings' or points of intra-corporeality include such matter.

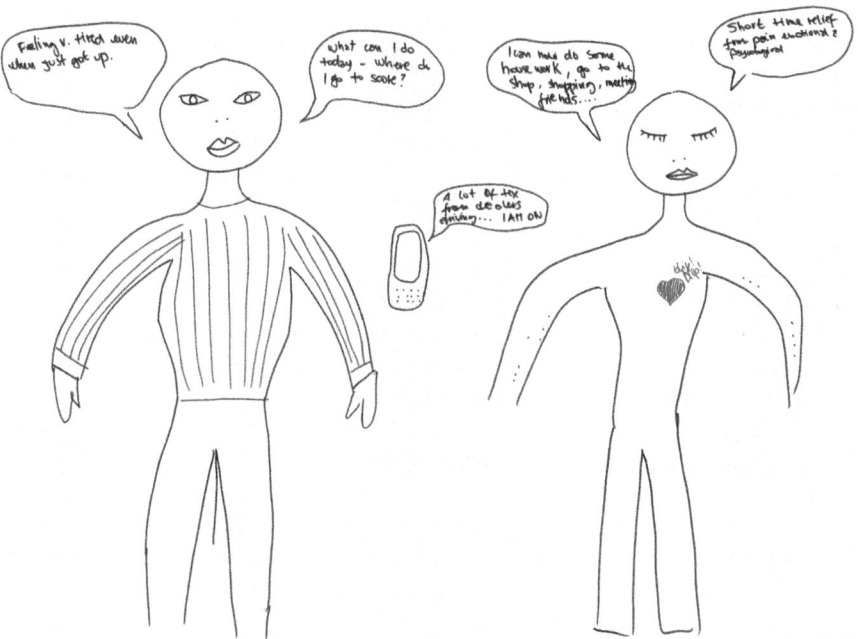

Figure 4.6 Silvie's body map. The mobile phone says: 'A lot of texts from dealers advertising ... I AM ON'.

Also, for Jon, whose body map (Figure 4.5) perhaps most starkly depicted some of these blockages in terms of a series of losses – his home, girlfriend, friends, families, cleanliness, nourishment – there is again a techno-corporal intra-action of bodies including the ATM (automated teller machine). The ATM and its declaration – 'you got nowt' – not only represented but stimulated a sense of abjection.

Similarly, in Mason and Mya's narratives, their addicted states were felt very much in relation to police bodies.

> You've constantly got that worry in the back of your mind, until you've got it in your body, basically, you're at risk of imprisonment so you know, that's a bit of a stress thinking about it. But you try not to think about it, cos you're just, if you think about it too much, paranoid and [worried the] police might pull me over, search me, which I think is a violation in itself. At the end of the day, if I want to medicate myself, I'll medicate myself.
>
> (Mason)

It is in these experiences with the police that his bad encounters materialise. It is the police that he tries not to think about rather than the substance, and it is in this haste to get the drug into his body that harm could be caused (Sarang et al., 2010). Mason feels that if he was able to use in a context of legalisation ('I wish it wasn't illegal'), these negative affects would be significantly reduced and heroin would have a better chance of remaining a good medication (helping him to cope with his difficult past) rather than a bad drug (that is able to put him in prison).

For Mya, it is not the drug that she is not living 'by choice' but the lack of control produced by its entanglement with police bodies and institutions who could 'chuck [her] out of society': 'that is the biggest reason why I stopped doing everything'.

> When you have to live it and you're not living it by choice, it doesn't become, it's very easy looking back on it and glamorizing it but when you're living it, it's not. You're constantly watching for the old bill, you know, the amount of times I've been in the middle of it and they've just totally picked me off the street and the next minute, I'm banged up for 3 years or banged up for 4 years. No, no, no, no. I don't want that again. It's not fun when the old bill can *chuck you out of society.* That is the biggest reason why I stopped doing everything, because if I go to prison again I'm going to *lose my house.* I'm going to have to start from rock bottom, I don't want that again. I just wanted out.

Although there is a physical sickness (made up of certain neurological chemicals interacting with the nervous system), this is always plugged into other bodies. It is in this connection with stratifying bodies that not only addiction is made but other harms arise, such as exploitation and losing one's home and liberty.

Lucy describes an assemblage of dealers, mobile phones, legal bodies, film images and gendered discourses, in which she is not only stratified as a drug user but also as a woman.

> Unless they, most dealers, they don't take it so they, it's just a business to them, so they don't give a monkey's [don't care] what happens to you what so ever. It's big money to them, whether you're sick is of no consequence to them. I mean that is what leads to a lot of incidences, sexual or not, because they know that you're desperate for something and they've got the power. And it's... the word pushing is for deal, because they've got a product and what it is, it's big money, they've got no consideration about ringing you or texting you constantly or going 'alright' in the street when you're with people, you know, it's happened to all of us, you know what I mean, or being sexual or whatever.

She really 'needs' the drugs (to remove withdrawal symptoms), but this cannot be separated from the other stratifying tendencies that connect her up to legal policies (illegality of drugs), images (objectivising women), dealers and mobile phones, in producing these power inequalities.

> If I take the conversations, especially in my 20s, you know, give us a blow job or do this and you can have what you want. If you don't have money don't worry about it, you know, you can have that... Absolutely vile [pause]. Somebody did it recently. He does it when I get tablets [Valium]. He goes 'oh yes, you come with me, you give me blow job, it'll be nice', and I'm just like 'no it's alright I'll give you the money', and I'm thinking I can't really afford this, it's costing me a fortune [pause]. I've got *something that you really need* and so I can use it [pause], make you work for it.

She goes on to highlight the role of films in trying to articulate these exploitable 'becomings', something that has also interested Vitellone (seen above), Malins (2004; 2009; 2011) and Fitzgerald (2015).

LUCY: I think that one of the best films about drugs is called 'Requiem for a Dream'.

FD: Oh yes.

LUCY: And that's exactly what it was like, that's exactly what it's like when a draught happens. It's horrific. And it's the worst thing that can happen and the lengths you have to go to, to get stuff, to get anything. I know it's American, but it's the most realistic one, it's the most realistic one on the way that things go.

FD: It's pretty….

LUCY: Grim. I know. And that's what I thought was better because… It's so realistic what that girl did, and it's so realistic what happened to that boy's arm, because that's much more likely than how they had *Trainspotting*, well the book was different, just going off with a load of cash, it isn't like that. It can take you to very dark places and destroy relationships and it's really horrible, and all for that needle, and the spoon, and the stuff, you know, just for that, all those people that just disappear and I think of all those sad faces (narrating her drawing) and just then, the people that you are seeing, it's just fake, there's so much fakeness.

It is in these assemblages that the power imbalances are emerge and form 'blocked becomings'. 'Of course, an assemblage of desire will include power arrangements (for example, feudal powers), but these must be located among the different components of the assemblage' (Deleuze, 1977: 132).

Following Malins (2004), these blockages are occurring not so much because of disorganisation (the 'sucked dry' BWO), but precisely because they are connected to too many stratifying (organising) bodies:

> Marginality arises through the particular stratifying tendencies of the various bodies of knowledge–such as medicine, law, psychiatry, public health, media, film, morality–that generally form part of the drug-assemblage.
>
> (2004: 90)

In this sense, discourses can be included as bodies, and concepts can be treated like 'things', which forms a 'radical constructivism'. This is particularly relevant in relation to the concept of the 'addict' and 'junkie'. Citing Deleuze, Henare et al. note:

> Discourse can have effects not because it 'overdetermines reality', but because no ontological distinction between 'discourse' and 'reality' pertains in the first place. In other words, concepts can bring about things because concepts and things just are one and the same (one and the same 'thing', we could say – using the term heuristically).
>
> (2007: 13)

Therefore, depending on the encounter, drug-using bodies can connect up with any number of different bodies and forces, including those which stratify these bodies as 'addicts', 'junkies' and 'women', and thus limit their ability to become-other. Although it is impossible to do full justice to the devastating ways these stratifications materialise, next I attempt to sketch out a few examples, including the ways participants describe having been blocked from becoming a party guest, boyfriend, employee and patient.

Blocked becoming...

... a party guest

In an event that massively affected Lucy, she recounts how the stigma of injecting heroin (being stratified as an addict by other guests), is, for her, far worse than any possible positive notion of the drug user image (like Carlos's 'bad boy' image). Unlike other party guests under the same circumstances (a missing purse), this stratification ('because of the association') immediately turned her into a thief rather than a guest, to the point that she felt unable to stay:

> The stigma can actually be more horrible, because, let me give you an example. There was a party and me and my boyfriend *were known*, and somebody couldn't find their purse and they went in my bag three times, ranting and raving, and then they found it in their car. So that part of it is really insulting. Because *they presume you're a thief all the time*. And it really made me upset, and I was really angry. I wouldn't steal off people. And it was a big family event on my boyfriend's side and his mum was stressed and there was loads of politics going on. *But because of the association*, because they know of our lifestyle, they... there was this panic and I remember just being so angry. I thought for fuck's sake, you've already been through my bag once, the accusation is such an insult.
>
> Then this person just rang up and said 'oh, I found my purse', and I just thought where's your bloody apology. And I just remember storming out and I remember just feeling so angry. I was so angry and so humiliated. Because there was this person ranting and raving around this place, and the image of... everyone was asked, but me and my boyfriend were asked too much, too intently, to the point that I just wanted to go, and I felt really tearful and... god the insults I've had to take.

There was a sense in Lucy's and other participants' accounts that people would try to treat them like non-drug users until something happened, and it was under this stress that the stratification intensified and cracks began to show (or erupt in Lucy's case). This bodily stratification is unsurprisingly felt at the somatic level, so that the 'humiliation' Lucy endured meant she no longer felt able to stay. The 'drug user' stratification also seemed to work in such a way that no apology was needed. Moreover, where this woman could rant and rave, Lucy just had to 'take' the insults, which meant subsuming them, internally. Lucy's becoming-other as a guest was squashed. She did not leave because of any closed-off desire to use drugs, as Deleuze might have predicted, but because her body – in being plugged into the junkie image of a thief – was no longer welcome.

In trying to explain further about the extent of this stratification, Lucy recounts another incident in which her boyfriend 'was wacked around the face by his stepmum and we were told that we should have labels put on us saying that we're dirty junkies'.

> There was a lot of politics going on because basically we were using and we were in a stage of moving house, and there was a lot of our stuff kept in their garden, but this box, where our needles were, were in this bag, really deep, and his father must have really gone in his cupboard and really gone to find them. So, he made this big deal about finding these pins in this box and then, they'd had a kid, and the boy wasn't very well, and I just remember the woman came storming through this kitchen and just wacked him. And she was American. And she was just screaming at us, saying *'you fucking junkies, you should wear a label, you don't bring that shit...'* there was just a lot of politics going on and a lot of upset because once it sort of gets out, a lot of families start saying it's his fault, or it's her fault, you caused it, nobody wants to say oh maybe that person's taking it *because they wanted to take it or because of the circumstances*, there's a lot of blame at the beginning. You're killing my son or you're killing my daughter, it's all your fault and you're an evil influence. Rather than, it's not like that, it's not people going 'hehe I want to make you a junkie', it just organically started to happen.

The syringes ('pins') are key to this story. In line with Vitellone's (2004; 2015) account explored in the last chapter, they do more than represent 'the junkie' but, in already being 'designated disgusting', produce affects and bodies, such as the 'junkie'. It is in finding the needles that the stepmother reacts in this way, and it is implied that she immediately links them to her son's illness. Mya also invokes this reaction: 'I mean there is a big stigma around injecting, I mean, hello, junkie, you use needles. We're the worst of the worst as far as society is concerned. It's not something you advertise, at all'. However, it is perhaps this very lack of advertising as Mya puts it that informs the stepmother's response. It was not clear that Lucy and her boyfriend were 'junkies' – their relationship to needles was not visible – and thereby this needed to be made visible through a label. It is hardly surprising that Lucy says there is nothing intentional about becoming a 'junkie' as this is a politically charged and negative effect of the drug encounter, which comes about in these connections with stratifying bodies – the media, public health, film, morality, etc. Being a 'junkie' or an 'addict' is not a physical state, but an involuntary and often oppressive sociomaterial one.

... a boyfriend

In another disturbing account of these blocked flows of desire, Matias recounts a story of how he was broken up from his girlfriend by being labelled a 'drug addict', even though he was not even using at the time.

MATIAS: I was doing the [university] course and I was living with my girlfriend, a Danish girl. She was a nurse. We were doing great, and I wasn't interested in drugs or anything, and my mum split us up, invited us for dinner for Christmas and then when we were at the table, she went in my girlfriend's handbag and got different numbers, her father, her sister, and started phoning them, telling them I was a drug addict and I was this and I was that.

FD: That's strange. Why was she doing that?

MATIAS: So she would split up with me.

FD: Was your partner using drugs as well?

MATIAS: No, no. And I was clean. But she wanted her family to tell her to leave me, and even though she didn't phone her father, she threatened to do it. And my girlfriend said 'no please don't do it, he has a heart condition, he might have a heart attack'. My mum said 'okay so move out of the flat'. So, we decided to split up for a while and we never got back together again. And I started using again.

Here, Matias could not escape from the association with drugs – the identity of a drug user – even though he had stopped using them. It was this unshakable identity that broke him and his girlfriend up. And, in the end, it was in this becoming-other being blocked that he returns to using drugs.

... an employee

In a long account which I feel is important to include in full, Sue recounts the way that she has been blocked from employment due to her criminal record as a drug user and sex worker. Even though she has long given up injecting (and has not smoked crack for many weeks), she continues to feel stigmatised and stratified as an 'addict' and 'prostitute'. It is in being prevented from becoming an employee that she feels inclined to 'fuck it' and start using again.

SUE: I'll show you something, I forgot I had this on me, I don't have to prove, I'm sure you believe me but this is my record (she shows me her Disclosure and Barring Service [DBS] record), look at the charges (about eighty for soliciting). They're on both sides, that's what I had to show at the job, and in the job, I was in the office, the recruitment office. These are all years ago – I was sixteen when I first got nicked. I got in a car in [north England] and they fucking caught me. The first car I got in. Cos in them days they used to nick you two or three times a night. They've never caught me talking to a man, just standing on the street you get arrested, if they know you as well.

FD: Is that still the case?

SUE: Yeah.

 (I look at the DBS)

SUE: There's a few drug ones.

FD: So this has caused a major problem in terms of getting jobs?

SUE: Well apparently, that woman who was at the agency... one of them works for my mum from that agency, so my mum kept phoning up so when she said, she already got the letter from the CRB (Criminal Records Bureau, now called DBS). Me, like an idiot, phoned her up and said I don't know if you'll take me on with my record. She said 'bring it in, you'll be alright'. I took it in, she went downstairs, said she'd gone to see the manager, and whilst she was down, women kept on coming up and looking at me. There was a room downstairs with women all on computers and they kept coming up and pretending, asking questions to the girl, then the two managers came up, called me into the back room, she said we're sorry but even if we send this to head office they'll say no. So I said okay, and just walked out. I was angry, but I didn't show it. I should have got them done for the way I was treated. They said if it was one page we would have taken you on but not twelve.

And I'd done all the training and everything. I had to go all the way to bloody East London, near A, you know, borrow money to get the bus fare up there every day. And then they told me no. And that put me off trying again [...] All I wanted was a job. And it's not good work care work; it's only £6 an hour. I just wanted to do something you know, to feel good inside, *instead of feeling dirty all the time,* it just fucking makes you feel like fuck it.

The DBS in this case is significant to the way Sue has been blocked from becoming an employee and continues to be stratified as a 'drug user' and 'prostitute', which gets felt at the level of the somatic body – she just wanted a job 'to feel good inside, instead of feeling dirty all the time'. It is in connection with the DBS, and the image of the 'junkie' and 'prostitute', along with the manager and other employees, that this stigmatised encounter (above) is created. And it is in being tied to these connections (in the DBS document) that limits Sue's potential to become-other. For some participants, the risks of these 'strata' or 'belts' following them into a life without drugs was even enough to put them off trying to abstain.

... a patient

Many participants recounted encounters in which they were blocked from becoming a 'worthy patient'. They felt stigmatised as drug users and felt they were given substandard treatment or even mistreated. Simon recalls a time when he suffered an overdose and was administered naloxone (an antidote that blocks opiate receptors) in hospital:

I felt sick immediately, obviously, and I said look I want to leave, I'm fine, I'm absolutely fine now, I want to leave, and they said no you can't, we're not going to let you, and I just tried to leave and I was putting on all my clothes and I wasn't being abusive or anything like that... And they just sent these fucking security guards, and there was four of these big heavy guys, and this is all on the CCTV, this was years ago, it's long gone now so perhaps I should forget about it, but I used to have asthma as a kid and they were like sitting on me and I was trying to say, with what breath I had left in my body, I'm honestly going in and out, I can't breathe. And they were all sitting on me like I was a criminal or something and I'd done something, like they were coppers [police].

This encounter has forcefully stayed with Simon ('perhaps I should forget about it') due to the severity of the response, its bodily imprint and the way it made him feel like a criminal. In being stratified as an addict, he was not treated like a patient, but as a criminal who could be restrained in this way. Matias also recalls a situation in which a senior doctor refused to treat him for gangrene from infected injection sites in his shoulders:

One of the doctors he said it was self-inflicted and he said yes let him go, and the other doctor, a younger doctor, was quite nice, and he said, this was in [hospital A], and he phoned [hospital B], and blah, blah, he arranged for me to be there at 9am the next day. And he said to me, it is very serious. I was studying medicine myself at university but I did only first year because of political problems I had to leave the country. The doctor says it is very serious, he explained, and I said I know. And I was there at 9am the next morning and they did everything, I was there for about a week and a half.

Many participants told similar stories of mistreatment, including experiences, when collecting their opiate substitute at pharmacies, of being ignored, treated with suspicion or having to wait until other customers had been served first.

Blocked but not stamped out

But the earth, or the body without organs, constantly eludes that judgement, flees and becomes destratified, decoded, deterritorialised.

Gilles Deleuze and Félix Guattari, 1987: 45

Following a Deleuzian ontology of desire, I have argued that becoming-with drugs takes many forms, including life sustaining and enhancing. Here, I have looked at how these connections also become blocked, but unlike some of Deleuze's (and with Guattari) thoughts on drugs, this does not appear to be because drug-using bodies are 'sucked dry' of organisation, but precisely the opposite, because they are exposed to too much organisation, that is, intra-acting social and material bodies. The addict is not a matter of the bounded drug-using body – the figure of the periwinkle in its shell – but a matter of encounter. Like with any other Deleuzian account of the body-without-organs, where there are encounters, there are also openings – a 'line of flight', or 'deterritorialisation'. That is, potentialities get blocked but not 'stamped out'. These 'power arrangements [...] continue to have repressive effect since they stamp out, not desire as a natural given, but the tips of assemblages of desire' (Deleuze, 1977: 15, my emphasis).

Assemblages are always caught in a dynamic of deterritorialisation and reterritorialisation. Therefore, although some becomings are blocked – a guest at a party, a boyfriend, an employee, a patient – and others become vulnerable, open to exploitation by dealers and a near-fatal overdose – there are still others getting made. Most defiantly, there is no 'turning point' to the extent that Deleuze argues, where vital connections become lethal connections. Indeed, even for Grigor, the participant in my study who appeared most blocked by his drug use ('my life is just no life really'), there were still connections being made and thus he felt it necessary, perhaps showing an awareness of pervading prejudices towards this life, that he did not want to die:

> But I'm so weak now that I've changed, you change, when you're on the drug you change, now I'm the bottom line. I'm not washing properly, haven't got my own place, so I'm staying at other peoples', staying on the floor, or couch or living room, I don't eat properly, I don't associate with people, I don't, *my life is just no life really*, I don't have a personal life, no nothing, I don't do any leisure or hobbies or – everything is gone, no relationship, no friendship, everything is gone. *Every day, every day just drugs*, and its everyday, as soon as I start and I can't stop until I don't have money. Cos I told you, the stuff is not very good, so even if I find the people with the best gear still I prefer dividing it into two because *I'm careful, I don't want to overdose.*

Grigor's account complies most strongly with the image of the disorganised addict, but still, this is relational. His addiction can be seen to be produced with the house he was living in and other people living there. This is where he positions the 'change'. He also says how this context means he cannot 'cold turkey' and begrudgingly has to rely on methadone:

> This is what I'm saying, it's changed (my drug use), because I even have to rely on the methadone to stop. Before I could say, I'm stopping and I'll do it cold turkey, like you know cold turkey, I've done it 3 or 4 times cold turkey by myself, not afraid of nothing. But now I don't have a place to stay, nothing, so I could do it cold turkey but I need to know I've got security, somewhere to stay, where I can lock the door and say

that's me, nobody's going to disturb me. But I don't have a place so now I have to rely on the medication to stop it, which I've never accepted.

As well as his dependency being felt as relational (with his housing situation), there was a sense that it was not linear (it ran no particular path towards disorganisation or 'loss of control'). Again, a loss of control seemed to be a matter of encounter rather than course. Hence, participants felt fed up when professionals expected a certain kind of deterioration towards a loss of control – a linear trajectory sometimes referred to as a drug-using career, where the drug user is seen to use drugs in increasing strength, frequency and combination, eventually, for those drawing of the Narcotics Anonymous model, 'hitting rock bottom'. Vicki therefore raises frustrations with doctors who assumed her status as a heroin user meant she was open to any drug going:

> And drink as well, even doctors, when you see doctors, they expect… they ask you over and over again if you use crack, if you drink and how much do you drink, and when you tell them no you don't… 'but how much?' 'NO NOT AT ALL!'. You know and it totally doesn't go in.
>
> (Vicki)

Reinforcing this idea that organisation is not lost, even when Vicki was using heroin daily, she made sure that her two friends and son ate well.

> For a couple of years things got hard again and the only thing I could usually get without money was gear, y'know, I mean I would always pay for it eventually, but… yeah, so we'd eat together, like to make it cheaper and I'd cook. We'd pay for it collectively and I'd do the cooking and the shopping usually. We used to eat quite well, we used to do quite well, living off special offers and reductions y'know. Feeding four people with £2.50, you become very resourceful.

So, to summarise, just because some drugs (mainly heroin) can cause a reliance with the genetic body, which materialise blockages in flows of desire (e.g. sickness), it is in their connection with other bodies (mobile phone, dealer, peers, needles, doctors) including those bodies with stratifying tendencies (connected to policies, knowledges, film and media images) that these negative effects are most prominently felt. But, as demonstrated, this does not mean that the body is 'sucked dry' of organisation and other connections cannot be made.

Conclusion

A body-in-becoming soon re-stratifies: either captured by, or lured by, the socius. Most often a drug using body is connected back up to the social machines of public health or medicine or morality through which it becomes stratified as a 'drug user' or 'addict' or 'deviant' respectively. Or the machine of law, through which it becomes stratified as a 'criminal' (or now, through diversionary programs: a 'recovering addict'!). Or it might, if we allow it, connect up to a multitude of other machines and become something else entirely (a student, an architect, a mother, a surfer, a masochist, a gardener, a knitter...).

Peta Malins, 2004: 88

I have used Deleuze's theory of desire and the body-in-becoming to make sense of participants' accounts of becoming-with drugs in terms of becoming-normal, -healthy, -other and -blocked. This challenges the body as a bounded object and instead further evidences the body-we-do. Bodies are desiring machines, that is, they are in constant connection with other bodies and gain their power to act or not therein. Addiction, along with other blockages such as illness, isolation, stigma and those associated harms, is a matter of encounter rather than inevitable course (or 'turning point'). So, when I asked Mya, 'So was it more to do with the grip that the drugs had over you?' it is perhaps by now no surprise that she responded with:

> *And the way of life.* You know, how can I get a methadone script when I'm not living nowhere, how can I get a doctor when I can't give no address. From when you're homeless, everything is against you. You can't get a doctor, you can't get a prescription, there's no way out. So you just go deeper and deeper into it.

It is not exclusively in connection to drugs that she experiences addiction (and blocked ways of becoming-other), but in these connections with other bodies – 'the way of life' – including the legal system, institutions, knowledges and policies, which mean she has no housing, doctor or prescription. It is through these connections that she went 'deeper and deeper into it', the 'periwinkle' in Deleuze's imagery. But in light of these accounts, this is the product of the drug encounter and assemblage. Therefore, unlike Deleuze, who foresees intervention at the 'turning point', I see it somewhere else: 'Why and how is this experience, even when self-destructive, but still vital, transformed into a deadly enterprise or generalized, unilinear dependence? Is it inevitable? *If there is a precise point, that is where therapy should intervene'* (Deleuze, 1978: 18).

This chapter has suggested that, rather than understanding drug use as running a unilinear course towards destruction, there is the co-existence of good and bad drug encounters, and thus we should be intervening to increase good connections, seen here in terms of becoming 'normal', 'healthy' and 'other', and decrease the bad, where lines of flight become blocked. This lends itself to a more intricate drug study and treatment based on a radical de-pathologisation of addiction as a matter of encounter.

In following this ontological shift in drug effects coming from innate and evil qualities to a matter of encounter, the next chapter problematises narrow ideals of recovering from such drugs. I will look at how participants' becomings with drugs, seen here, and in Chapters 2 and 3, can be better understood as habit, and, like others have argued, how this could offer the 'otherwise' necessary for a more caring intervention grounded in people's more-than-human relationality, as opposed to trying to, often violently, break such vital connections. As Malins succinctly expresses: 'We all need our desiring outlets, otherwise we rigidify and die'. These care practices, based on making new habits and desiring connections, move us towards alternative ways of thinking and intervening with drugs.

Notes

1 Heroin when smoked is placed on a line of aluminium foil, lit from underneath and 'chased' along its length. Smokers may have to do this several times over to get the same effects as an injection, and hence why it is understood as time-consuming. Where the effects of an injection can last several hours, smoking heroin has to be repeated throughout the day, which is problematic for people who work, or simply do not wish to take up vast amounts of their day using substances. It also releases an odour, which would be detectable, and thus dictates where people can be, for example, not at work.

2 Drug Rehabilitation Requirements are community orders issued to people who use drugs, intended to reduce their drug use and the associated criminal activity. They are ordered to attend treatment and regular drug testing and can be imprisoned if in breach of the order.

Chapter 5

Intervening-with bodies

Troubling recovery: mediating habits and doing more-than-harm reduction

> The government recognises we must go further than merely reducing the harms caused by drug misuse, and offer every opportunity for people to *choose* recovery as a way out of dependency.
>
> Home Office, 2012: 6, my emphasis

> They put you in a rehab for like a couple of weeks for a habit that's been twenty years in the making.
>
> Nadiya, 44 years old, injects heroin

In this book thus far, we have looked at the multiple bodies involved in injecting drug use, which problematises the idea that drugs have casual effects and are individually chosen for these effects. This is not to say there is a loss of control, but to develop an understanding of agency that no longer requires such binaries as 'out of/in control'. A wider disruption has also taken place, challenging our bifurcated world, which has shaken-up a reliance on other dichotomies such as addiction/freedom, mind/body and individual/environment, and thus liberated how we can think *with* and *do* drugs differently. In this chapter, I want to consider how these relational bodies reimagine a vision of recovery implemented in UK service provision.

Although a move towards abstinence-based drug treatment can be traced to the turn of the century (Stimson, 2000), a shift to recovery was intensified in the period leading up to and during my fieldwork. The 2010 Drug Strategy ratified abstinence-based recovery as the defining feature of UK drug treatment in its title: Reducing Demand, Restricting Supply, *Building Recovery:* Supporting People to Live a *Drug Free Life* (Home Office, 2010, my emphasis). The Strategy marked a shift from previous governments' attention on harm reduction (MacGregor, 2017). Volunteering at the Dunswell service in 2013, and returning in 2014 for the research, I witnessed these transitions and the shift in focus from supporting service users to *manage* their illicit drug use (without necessarily abstaining), along with their substitute medication (ensuring the dose is preventing withdrawals) and daily lives (with health, social, economic, psychological issues) to more forcefully encouraging service users to end their drug use as the key solution to their problems. Consequently, it is perhaps no surprise that this narrower conception of drug use as in need of ending rubbed up against the relationality of bodies and their contingent effects I encountered in the interviews, drawings and observations with people who inject/use drugs. However, troubling recovery yet further, given our onto-epistemological entanglements, it can be implicated in producing the very 'blockages' it intends to relieve or 'unstick', to use a common term employed in the recovery discourse (below). The recovery agenda, for example, was intimately involved in one participant's 'internal conflicts' as he tried to distance himself from his desire for drugs, and other harms were potentialised as participants found themselves ill understood at services privileging abstention. Indeed, for some commentators, this has even initiated a fatal connection as the numbers of those in treatment have fallen and drug-related deaths have soared (ACDM, 2016; Boyt, 2014; Hamilton and Stevens, 2017; 2018). It is more important than ever that we trouble these recovery discourses and practices to allow for the complexities in peoples' drugged experiences.

To do so, this chapter takes three parts. First, I develop a notion of becoming-with drugs (seen in the previous chapters) as habit, which, building on the work of others in the field, offers an 'otherwise' to addiction and dependency. It accounts for but is not reducible to a physical dependency, and, as such, is always located beyond 'the body' (e.g. brain). As a common term used by participants and drug users more widely, I want to take habit seriously, beyond a colloquialism for addiction, and explore what this may achieve for thinking, doing and intervening with drugs differently. Habit, unlike addiction, can take seriously the repetition in drug use patterns whilst also allowing for the differences that escape it. To repeat the language of the last chapter, growth is not stamped out. Second, I will use this notion of becoming-with drugs as habit to trouble an enactment of recovery based on an anterior relationship between bodies (e.g. the user and drug).

'Trouble', following Haraway, is used here both as a verb, to denote a diffractive style of analysis that refuses to be led by *a priori* binaries, and a noun for describing our dystopian anthropocentric world. Wanting, as I have said, to 'stay with the trouble' (to not simplify or shy away from the magnitude of problems that are always moving and in tension), I look at how a notion of habit can question recovery strategies based on breakable divides between the user and drug, mind and body, past and present, and what is considered internal (e.g. will) and external (e.g. 'triggers'). In the third part of the argument, I consider how, at the same time as these reductive enactments of recovery are occurring, they are becoming unsettled. Service providers worked within sociomaterial collectives to 'fiddle with' recovery technologies and modes of knowing to enact alternative treatment approaches based on bodies-as-habit in resisting both recovery and harm reduction models in practicing what one service provider called 'harm reduction and *more*'.

Becoming-with drugs as habit

> I think everything, from making phone calls to the dealers, to going to buy, everything is psychological, you get *used* to that, you know, it's not just like doing [the drugs], *it's the whole thing*, it's very addictive, the whole thing, I don't know, it's *becoming part of your daily life*. I don't know whether the brain gets used to it, I don't know, because ever if you stop doing it, then *you're missing* the phone calls, going to the place, coming back, opening the ... you know, everything ... *It's not just about the drug it's about the whole* ... Some people think it's only about the drugs, no I don't think so. We're all different so people experience it in different ways, I'm sure. I can only say what I think from myself. But it's not just about, because, for me, if I stayed at home and somebody bring it for me, I would miss that part of going out and... but because I'm used to going by myself all the time, maybe that's what I'm used to, maybe somebody else, the boyfriend goes for them so they don't know, they don't miss that part, do you know what I mean? So it's about how you see it, *how you get used to it*.
>
> Silvie, 44 years old, injects 'speedballs'

> Habit [...] is the link that bridges the relations between the organic and the inorganic, introducing the needs of the organism to its environment and inserting its environment into the behaviour of the organism.
>
> Elizabeth Grosz, 2013: 234

Silvie is drawing attention to the fact that her drug use is about more than the substance: 'It's not just about the drug, it's about the whole...' It's about the 'calls to the dealers', 'going to buy', 'coming back', 'opening the [drug bags]'. It is this that becomes part of her 'daily life', which she has become 'used to', and would 'miss' if she was to stop. The outer and inner worlds become enmeshed. Habit as a kind of affect modulation is intriguing because it is just as much about process and change as the marks it leaves. Habit is where the past makes an imprint on the present and future, where the external world enters the internal, and where everyday rhythms and speeds get under the skin. Paradoxically, habit operates according to movement through stasis (Deleuze, 1994; Deleuze and Guattari, 1994). That is, by the past enacting the present, the present is already changed, enacting the future. In this sense, habit is fundamentally about process. 'Habit draws something new from repetition – namely, difference' (Deleuze, 1994: 73). So, for Silvie, habit is far from constant. She allows for such differences in drug habits, for example, if 'the boyfriend goes for them so they don't know, they don't miss that part...we're all different so people experience it in different ways'. This is a much more open understanding of repetition than that found in the neurological concept of addiction (Dilkes-Frayne et al., 2017; Pienaar and Dilkes-Frayne, 2017; Pienaar et al., 2017). Here, I want to build from the previous chapters on becoming-with drugs to add to an already established discourse on understanding regular drug use as habit in order to support its currency as a productive otherwise to addiction or dependency. Indeed, in the third part of the chapter, I consider how habit is already being 'machined' in care practices as service providers speak to the situatedness of people's needs and desires to help them channel, through their relationality, new, 'healthier' habits.

'Machinic habit'

As we have seen throughout the book, bodies are always in a state of becoming of which drugs can be a part. Where addiction models can be seen to enact a body-we-have – a classical account of the bounded objective body, owned by a mindful subject (in the twelve-step models, one never overcomes addiction, but remains in control of it through daily mental work) – habit allows an engagement with the body-we-do, firmly in flux. Like others (Fraser, 2016; Fraser et al., 2014; Keane, 2002; Valverde, 1998), I follow here Eve Sedgwick's proposal for habit as an 'otherwise' to addiction:

> I'll just suggest briefly that the best luck I've had so far in reconstructing an 'otherwise' for addiction attribution has been through a tradition that is, not opposed to it or explanatory of it, but rather one step to the side of it. That is the tradition of habit, a version of repeated action that moves, not toward metaphysical absolutes, but toward interrelations of the action – and the self-acting – with the bodily habitus, the apparelling habit, the sheltering habitation, everything that marks the trace of that habit on a word that the metaphysical absolutes would have left vacuum.
> (Sedgwick, 1993: 138)

I draw also from a special edition on habit in the journal, *Body & Society* (Bennett et al., 2013). In this issue, Grosz (2013) observes that 'philosophical reflection may be able to provide another angle on habits'. In light of this, I draw on habit through Bergson-Deleuze and Spinoza-Deleuze (amongst others, such as, William James and Gabriel Tarde) as seen, for example, in the work of Blackman (2013), Grosz (2013), Latour (2013) and Massumi (2015), in relation to bodies that move as they feel and feel as they move, learning to become affected as they go along. I wish here to explore habit as a way of understanding how participants' drug practices and experiences are materially entangled within the body, which makes any simple idea of separating the body from the substance problematic.

The 'habit' put forward in Silvie's account and seen throughout in participants' drug-using practices is different from some of the traditional ways habit has been dealt with in the drug and addiction field. Habit has been conceptualised as a fixed mechanical behaviour in addiction psychology, a construct of neoliberal governmentality, and a matter of embodied action tied to wider social and economic structures through Pierre Bourdieu's concept of habitus. Governmentality theory has been particularly useful in exploring the ways that good habits have been encouraged and bad habits (like drug use, and, in particular, injecting) have been worked on and adjusted through various disciplining techniques (Dodsworth, 2013), such as methadone programmes (Bourgois, 2000; Fraser and valentine, 2008), needle exchanges (McLean, 2011) and supervised injecting clinics (Fischer et al., 2004). Bourdieu's work on habitus has also offered much insight into the complex intersection between structure and individual behaviour (e.g. Bourgeois and Schonberg, 2009; Parkin, 2013). However, here, I tap into a recent interest in forms of agency that by-pass reason and disrupt a metaphysics of being in the 'turn to affect' (Clough and Halley, 2007). That is, the habits observed in this study speak to Massumi's (2002) concept of machinic habit, which can be distinguished from human habit or habitus, as a 'machining' of more-than-human drug-using or injecting bodies through affect modulation.

Machinic habit is a form of bodily memory, residing at the intersection of inner and outer worlds. Habit is central to how people learn to be affected and affect, for (as already seen) 'pleasure', 'vitality', 'normality', 'health' and 'otherness'. This has been extremely helpful in understanding participants' drug use in a way that can take their practices more seriously. Habit is more than a physical dependency but a matter of drug-body-world entanglement. And, as such, it is no coincidence that participants here, and drug users more widely, tend to refer to themselves as having a habit rather than an addiction, or, at least, in addition to an addiction. Where addiction is narrow in its focus, habit allows for wider patterns of embodiment. For example, Simon says:

> I do see it as a habit, there is a lot about getting up, getting to the time that they [drug dealers] switch on, going out and getting the stuff and coming back and having a... you know, having a use, that's, a lot of that is habit, just cos *it's what I do* [...] It's a funny, it's a very strange relationship, you do almost feel, there is a quality where it's almost like a friend, you know, that it's quite comforting sometimes, the feeling is very comforting.

Simon explains that a lot of his drug using is a habit. It is what he *does*. There is a momentum in his voice to the rhythms of this work: 'there is a lot about getting up, getting to the time that they switch on, going out and getting the stuff and coming back and having a... you know, having a use'. Like with Silvie, the process of scoring is seen to be just as integral to the using itself, which is perhaps overlooked in drug studies that tend to focus on the injecting practice (e.g. for public health studies, where blood-borne virus vulnerability is located). Simon brings to our attention how habits have become part of him – a new way of being-in-the-world – which, as suggested throughout the book, makes it hard to give up. This alludes to Massumi's idea that habit is integral to individuating, where people are *made* in processes of sociomaterial assembling. For Fraser and valentine (2008), drawing on Hacking's concept of 'making up people', methadone clients get constituted 'as unreliable and immature, in need of moral guidance'. Bodies are governed and disciplined through treatment as a form of 'biopower', which includes the role of metaphor, such as 'liquid handcuffs', to enact these 'constrained subjects' (2008: 117–19). And in Carr's ethnography, addiction treatment is seen 'as a site where ideologies of language are refined and reproduced, processing people along the way' (2011: 233). Here, I consider the way people are made with habits as a matter of affect modulation and thus as integral to *embodiment*. That is, in following Massumi's reading of Spinoza:

> What a body is, he says, is what it can do as it goes along. This is a totally pragmatic definition. A body is defined by what capacities it carries from step to step. What these are exactly is changing constantly. A body's ability to affect or be affected – its charge of affect – isn't something fixed.
>
> (Massumi, 2015: 4)

Habits change our capacity to affect and be affected, and thus precede individuation: 'Habits contract to form me. That's taking "me" to be the relational matrix of reactivation that my body carries forward – which *is* my body as I defined it before. "My" comes before "me"' (Massumi, 2015: 65, original emphasis).

This concept of habit is concerned with the everydayness of life, which affects us all – how we are constantly becoming sensitised *with* the world. In this sense, the speeds involved in the routines and habits of drug use – the scoring, cooking up, injecting – are materially embedded in the way participants come to individuate.

> …there is a pure plane of immanence, univocality, composition, upon which everything is given, upon which unformed elements and materials dance that are distinguished from one another only by their speed and that enter into this or that *individuated assemblage depending on their connections, their relations of movement.*
>
> (Deleuze and Guattari, 1987: 255, my emphasis)

However, there is a paradox, just as movement seems to get locked into bodies, new movement is created. As rhythms get made and become imprinted they become unmade – there is always difference in repetition. Or, as Deleuze says, 'difference inhabits repetition' (1994: 76). This is an inherently more optimist approach than addiction and gets drawn to our attention in Nadiya's account.

> To me, I think the most of it would be, I think, if you had 100% of all these things that you asked, I think habit would take about 75%, it's just something, it's like smoking cigarettes, they're bad for you but then you know you wake and you, I see people on the TV wake up and light up and I think what the fuck, it just reminds you. I think if you stop, when you wake up in the morning it'll be the first thought, but about two or three weeks down the line, you wake up some mornings and you won't think about it, you know, you'll think about something else. A lot of time needs to pass for you to stop, and I think that's the worst part because in the meantime, you've got really nothing to do, and people aren't really going to take up menial jobs or I don't know. It's a vicious cycle.

Although Nadiya points to a vicious cycle much like the spiralling black holes in Deleuze and Guattari's imagery, this is by no means beyond change. She explains that her drug use is mainly about habit as opposed to addiction – 'if you had 100 per cent of all these things [habit, addiction, dependency] that you asked, I think habit would take about 75 per cent'. One can assume these are the habits of getting up, going to get the drug, using and everything in-between that has occupied her daily routines and rhythms for nearly ten years. Therefore, she says that in changing those patterns, in not doing this, she can change her desire for drugs – 'but about two or three weeks down the line, you wake up some mornings and you won't think about it, you know, you'll think about something else'. There is the potential for something different. Nevertheless, this is no easy task and she cautions: 'a lot of time needs to pass for you to stop'. However, crucially, for this to happen, she needs something else to *do* to pass the time. To reiterate from other parts of the book, time is thus not an abstract phenomenon (an objective measure), but reliant on what we do and the 'things' used to navigate its passing, topologically.

Machinic habit allows for repetition and change, and, as alluded to in the book's Introduction, it is this repetition that is sometimes missed in other post-human and actor-network theory (ANT)-influenced accounts of drug use that focus on tracing 'things' rather than what moves us between and beyond them (Dilkes-Frayne and Duff, 2017). Therefore, next, I will spend some time exploring how, in an ontology of process, habits manage to stick.

Habit's 'sticking point'

> The question that such [process] ontological models raise is how some force of order, some process of stabilization, may wrench from the

turbulence of these forces of differentiation a measure of rest, a kind of cohesion or unity, a continuity over time.

Elizabeth Grosz, 2013: 230

In a world in-becoming, how do certain habits stick? How is it possible for participants to want to repeat certain processes when every event is somehow starting anew or rather has never ended? How is it that participants desire and sometimes unknowingly find themselves pursuing the processes of going out to score, going through the necessary preparatory practices to find a vein, using drugs and, for some, almost immediately using again, sometimes without barely knowing what they are doing? For example, in reference to drinking her methadone, Suzy says:

> I wake up every morning, and I've got the methadone in my draw next to my bed, and before I've even engaged my brain, I've poured it out, and gone 'glug' (she demonstrates this drinking action).

How and where do these memories reside? But, also, where do these habits slip? These are the points that highlight Deleuze's paradoxical notion that it is in these bodily memories that change occurs. A philosophy of immanence is about change, but, for change, there needs to be moments of repetition, and this is how habit comes to play a central role in a theory of process.

> But for [Deleuze], difference, divergence, variation, elaboration also requires repetition, never sameness or identity, but generative repetition and its creative forms, contraction, synthesis or habit.

(Grosz, 2013: 231)

Habit is not about stasis or being 'stuck' (to use a word, as I said, commonly employed in drug services, to be taken up further below), rather, by habits holding bodily memories of the past, they are inherently changing the future. Latour calls habit the 'most indispensable' mode of existence: 'the one that takes up 99 percent of our lives, the one without which we could not exist' (2013: 264). For Grosz, habit is 'a fundamentally creative capacity that produces the possibility of stability in a universe in which change is fundamental' (2013: 219). Habits form our routines and speeds that bring the outer world inside, and past into the present, which makes change possible and in Bergson's account frees up thought. Therefore, just because there is a habit does not mean there is a lack of relatively free acts or thought. In fact, for Bergson and Deleuze, it makes such radical thinking possible:

> Bergson cites the familiar reaction we have to an alarm clock early in the morning, part of the habitual routine of each work-day [e.g. Suzy's glug of methadone]. The alarm summons up a chain of actions: opening

our eyes, turning off the alarm, getting out of bed, putting on slippers and beginning the day. It is only because we undertake these activities in a state of half-consciousness that we have the energy and interest to undertake less routinized actions, to elaborate relatively free acts. Habits, incorporating memories of past performances in similar contexts, leave both consciousness and the energetic forces of the body able to address other issues than the habitual only because the habitual accommodates so much of what is required from us.

(Grosz, 2013: 226)

Habits are central to life and thereby where I talk about habits this should not be thought of as necessarily restraining bodies. Indeed, habit 'comes into the present as an inheritance of the past, but only to the extent that it is readying a future' (Massumi, 2015: 59).

Habits are central to how we do our bodies and become embodied. This is not about how a body and 'thing' (e.g. drug) interact, but how they change each other and thus are also existing beyond each other. This helps to explain why, in processes of habit, affects can circulate beyond a causal effect. Where drug addiction requires a drug, habit is about how bodies become-with drugs, so, for some participants, affects could be actualised without the drug itself being consumed.

> Yeah, and I suppose it's just got a habit, like ritual sort of thing, like cooking it up, you start getting the feelings like you've already had it when you haven't.
>
> (Crystal)

The habit for Crystal is linked to this expansion in affect, where the repetition of action means that her body feels the affects 'like you've already had it when you haven't'. The 'sticking point', rather than being in the flesh (e.g. in neurological transmitters) resides elsewhere in that moment. Similarly, Meg explains how the positive drug effects associated with heroin exist beyond its administration: 'Once you've got it in your hand you start to feel better, as soon as you've got it'. Resonating with this, but to the opposite effect, Tom describes how just having the drug in his possession can cause withdrawals:

> as soon as you get back, even if you're fine, even if I've done my methadone and I feel fine [...] as soon as I get back and I've got a bag [of heroin], I'll start getting withdrawal symptoms, I'll start feeling nauseous and stuff like that, just because I know I'm about to relieve it.

In these accounts of habit, drug effects are no longer causally locked into matter. It is through a similar observation that Deleuze and Guattari go even further to suggest that the drug experimentation may not need the substance at all:

> Could what the drug user or masochist obtains also be obtained in a different fashion in the conditions of the plane, so it would even be possible to use drugs without using drugs, to get soused on pure water, as in Henry Miller's experimentations?
>
> (1987: 166)

Habit is central to the production of affects and therefore it is perhaps not surprising that the practices associated with injecting drugs were often thought about as being of equal, if not, more importance to the substance itself.

> I think *you get used to feeling* like that, and when you, when you go back to smoking, it kind of, *you don't feel it,* it takes a while to get back to that, you know, you need to completely stop injecting and then you have to get used to smoke again, it's not like, you can't just say, one day I'm smoking, do you know what I mean? If you're used to injecting and then you smoke, one day, you don't feel it, you need so much to feel the same, unless you're stopping and slowly get used to.
>
> (Silvie)

For some participants, as I have already drawn attention to in Chapter 3, the preparatory practices and route of administration were so vital for the desired effects that they would rather not use heroin if it was not injected or use crack and heroin together if it was not 'speedballed'.

But, as also seen, even though habits become firmly embedded, they are not beyond change. The issue, as highlighted by Nadiya, is not that new habits cannot be made, but that making new habits takes time (again, where time is relational). Drawing again on Nadiya's account of habit above, she indulges me in a discussion of what habit could offer as an otherwise to addiction. I will quote this dialogue in full to try and do service to the nuance in her account, before thinking more about what it could suggest.

FD: So it's not necessarily that it's a whole thought process going on, it's just something that you've got used to doing?

NADIYA: It's just like smoking [cigarettes] really, but you know obviously more expensive and bad for you, I think they're both bad for you though, cos smoking…

FD: I'm interested in the body and embodied feelings, so for me it's quite interesting that it's not necessarily a conscious thing, it could be the body…?

NADIYA: I don't think that is necessarily true, I think a lot of this thing is to do with your mental state. The body is only when you're withdrawing, when your body is telling you, that's when the body is speaking to you, but everything else is to do with a mental thing. It's a mental thing because it's constantly on your mind, and it will be even more so when you're withdrawing, you know. Actually a friend of mine said when you're sick and somebody brings you something, it's as if they brought you a hundred doctors, that's you know, because then it just stops, this horrible physical feeling that you get.

FD: But the thoughts of wanting to use, it's not like thoughts that you're consciously thinking, or is it something you're in control of?

NADIYA: No, it's not conscious thinking about it. It's definitely subconscious. *Everything is pulling you*, again it's not physical, it's mental, this pull, but it definitely exists.

FD: The pull. And would you say that your drug use is something that you're in control of?

NADIYA: No, I don't think anybody is, and whoever said they are, they're lying.

FD: Well I suppose it could depend on the drug?

NADIYA: Well, still, there's a lot of people that say the same thing. Well actually it's not true, a lot of people like to think so, but you know if you said okay let's not do it for a month, they wouldn't be able to do it. Cos I've actually challenged a few who are just smokers (cigarettes), and they wouldn't be able to do it for a week let alone a month... And these are all *habitual things, really mental things.* I don't know maybe alcoholics get the physical withdrawal as well from alcohol. A lot of people who started on heroin became alcoholic, basically, I know a lot of them, you know, most of them actually who had a heroin habit. Kicked it for like not a few weeks, like six months in a rehab. They're all now full-blown alcoholics now. I don't know really what's worse. *They put you in a rehab for like a couple of weeks for a habit that's been twenty years in the making.*

In this excerpt, I follow up on Nadiya's account of habit by letting her know that this resonates with my interests in the body. However, she is quick to disagree: 'I don't think that is necessarily true, I think a lot of this thing is to do with your mental state. The body is only when you're withdrawing'. But, it appears, as the conversation moves on, we might actually be talking about the same thing. I think she is highlighting that addiction is about more than the biological body, which she sees as involved 'only when you're withdrawing'. This connects to modes of thought on the difference between physical and psychological addiction, where heroin is seen as physically addictive, but something like crack cocaine is seen as 'psychologically addictive' (a distinction widely made in addiction discourse and in drug services). Nadiya is trying to complicate this divide in highlighting that there is more to heroin use than the physical addiction. 'Everything else is to do with a mental thing. It's a mental thing because it's constantly on your mind'. But, this is also more than an account of 'psychological addiction': this is more than conscious thought, rather, she says, 'everything is pulling you'. In exploring further, this 'pull' seems to be associated with habit, and by talking about the 'mental' side, she is talking about habit: 'these are all habitual things, really mental things'. And it is the habit of using drugs, like, she says, with cigarettes and alcohol that people find hard to give up, and thus many people she knows have come to replace one habit with another. Again, this disrupts an account of substances in terms of their essences: the substance itself is less important than the habit. Thus, Nadiya makes an astute observation: 'They put you in a rehab for like a couple of weeks for a habit that's been twenty years in the making'. This for me sums up a lot of the difficulties that my interlocutors (service users and providers) found with a reductionist application of the recovery agenda in which habits are not taken seriously. Before exploring this further in the following section, I will attend more closely to a notion of 'triggers' that calls habit to eventful attention.

'Triggers': calling habit to eventful attention

The whole ritual becomes addictive. The needle fixation, the whole getting everything out, there's lots of senses that affect you psychologically and physically. It's amazing. Even a voice I'm hearing on the phone, I could be feeling alright and then suddenly I'm pouring with sweat. And cos... say for instance if I'm at work and I'm feeling alright for a bit, and then as soon as he mentioned it, I'd just be pouring with sweat and feel like we've got to go and get something. It's incredible how psychosomatic, how powerful that is... It's like mad, like when I've been on the train to the coast, and as soon as I've started coming back into London, this panic seems to come on. And, where I've coped with the texts and messages with people (drug dealers), you know, being 'on' (available), I've just gone, ahh, I've got to get to the station. I've got to go to the station. I've got to get onto the train. Even now, it's amazing... people go "are you alright", you're just pouring with sweat all down your back.

Lucy, 42 years old, injects heroin

[Triggers] call habit to eventful attention. They impinge with force. They impact. They arrive, and insist (on the practical impossibility of their own systemic envelopment). [Triggers are] the transformational callback to feeling of the so-automatic as to be ignored.

Brian Massumi, 1998: 156

In replacing Massumi's word 'sensation' with 'triggers', we can see how triggers could easily be imagined as feelings arising from where bodies have become habituated. Triggers call attention to these inscriptions that are hard to articulate but draw us in nonetheless. We need to start taking triggers seriously in order to recognise the nonconscious aspects of drug use frequently overlooked in sociological research (historically favouring the rational individual), without reducing the phenomenon to 'addiction', which only too readily omits complexities (see Dennis, 2016). Lucy describes some of the senses involved in these situations which bring about her desire to use heroin. She elaborates on the 'senses that affect [her] psychologically and physically' in describing a feeling of panic as she comes back to London. It is clear to Lucy that what informs her heroin use goes beyond (without necessarily excluding) a rationally chosen reason to use, but rather is intimately related to her environment. In particular, she names the role of text messages, mobile phones, certain words, voices, bodies and space.

Drawing out the role of words and the space-time configuration of London, Lucy comments:

> So, the word 'on' is such a big, that's all it has to say, 'on', which means he's on, just that word and it's, you know, it's so powerful...

The word 'on' moves her. This chimes with how bodies, in Latour's account of learning to become affected by the perfume training kit, become sensitised to words:

> Once we have gone through the training session, the word 'violet' carries at last the fragrance of the violet and all the chemical undertones. Through the materiality of the language tools, *words finally carry worlds*.
> (2004a: 210, my emphasis)

Habits could also be tied to specific space-times such as London, and thus desires to use drugs were most acutely felt when in these connections.

> If I'm seeing my dad, it's in my head. I leave my phone in my bedroom at my dad's, so I can keep my head out of it. But in [London], as soon as that text comes through, I start thinking about it straight away.
> (Lucy)

> I come back from seeing my daughter from outside London, I take enough tablets, wean myself down, get back to London and [...] the minute you see it you'll want it, it's very difficult.
> (Gwen)

As Massumi says, 'it takes you, before you have it as your memory. It catapults you into unfolding tendency before any possibility of reflection' (2015: 59). Triggers are affective energies that get left behind in encounters between the body and environment in drug-using events, directing or 'machining' bodies in their flows of desire. That is, Lucy and Gwen are moved by these previously assembling things, forces and bodies, rather than any unique object or subject ('the trigger'). This means that they may do their best to avoid these encounters, but these habituated channels can compel them – 'as soon as the text comes through' or 'the minute you see it, you'll want it'.

Having established habit as a way of thinking about how bodies become-with drugs as an otherwise to addiction, I now wish to attend to how this troubles UK drug policy based on the 'full recovery' of an individual with a drug problem, which became increasingly influential during fieldwork, and, as I observe, narrowly defined. This section again takes a layered approach. First, I will outline the recovery agenda. Second, I will show how it was enacting a restrictive kind of movement towards abstinence, with a particular focus on methadone. Third, I will suggest some harms that might be ensuing.

'The recovery agenda'

> In terms of the recovery agenda [...] people are pushing for drug-free completion rates, you have to be drug-free, so people aren't getting paid for people *in treatment,* you're getting paid for people *leaving treatment.*
> (Eva, recovery worker, Dunswell service)

The 2010 Drug Strategy (Home Office, 2010), *Reducing Demand, Restricting Supply, Building Recovery: Supporting People to Live a Drug Free Life,* marked a substantial shift in UK drug policy. Known as the recovery agenda by the participants in this study, it moved away from previous harm reduction emphases towards a more abstinence-focussed treatment system. 'Harm reduction', a once defining concept of UK drug policy, particularly as a public health response to HIV/AIDS in the 1908s and 1990s (Stimson, 2007), was not mentioned in the 2010 Drug Strategy (Home Office, 2010), a trend which continues in the most recent drug policy (Home Office, 2017). Instead, *'full recovery'* became the target for drug service delivery. Underpinned by metrics governing the performance (and thus funding) of drug services in relation to this target, 'full recovery' constitutes treatment as abstinence from all substances, including prescribed substitution medications (Home Office, 2010; 2012; National Health Service, 2012). The 2012 'roadmap' (Home Office, 2012), *Putting Full Recovery First,* outlined how drug services should be restructured in line with these abstinence goals, with the explicit intention to 'shake up the maintenance oriented status quo of heroin addiction' – a vision and call to arms that we see being implemented below. Furthermore, in the National Health Service (NHS, 2012) report, *Medications in Recovery: Re-orientating Drug Dependence Treatment,* opiate substitution treatment (OST) is specifically redefined as a recovery technology. These new policies ignited a wave of evangelism about the promise that recovery might afford (Home Office, 2012; Lancaster et al., 2015; McKeganey, 2012; Monaghan, 2012).

Service providers, including managers and workers, draw extensively on the metaphor of movement in describing recovery and the imagery of stasis of which it escapes. Eva, a recovery worker (by the time of my return to the service in 2014, all drug workers had been renamed recovery workers) at the Dunswell service, says: 'Now it's about the *movement,* the through-puts or whatever, of people coming through the system and out the other side'. The recovery agenda is seen to be about getting people *through* treatment as opposed to what is characterised by some as a harm reduction approach based on 'keeping them safe' *in* treatment. And not only that, it could enact a 'rapid' movement:

> So the recovery agenda is [...] the idea that clients can *move forward rapidly* [...] it's like from, you know, from the onset you're looking at a client and saying how do you want to plan your recovery? How long?
>
> (Simone, project leader, Dunswell service)

This 'movement' is supported by a change in monitoring and the way drug services are funded. Although 'payment-by-results' had not been fully implemented in either of the services in the study, workers spoke of a 'payment by results in kind' in which services were increasingly paid according to whether service users had achieved a drug-free successful completion rather than for the service they had provided.

Engaging with movement as more than a metaphor but as an ontology or rather multiple ontologies, something else is going on, which holds promise for an alternative treatment approach based on desire and machining habits (as oppose to giving them up). I will now look at the two possible ways that movement may be getting enacted. The first relies on a movement towards abstinence, where drug users, on the flip side, have become 'stuck'. The drug therefore becomes the focus of attention, the habit that needs to be broken, to become 'unstuck'. Controversially, this too can include substitution medication and thus methadone becomes a rallying point for this stasis – people are said to be 'parked' on it and 'stuck' in treatment (CSJ, 2013; 2014). Bodies that can be moved in this way towards abstention – those with other social, material, economic support or flows of desire to plug into – become privileged or 'cherry picked' over those that cannot. Therefore, those service users who are less able to be moved in these ways – to live a life free of, namely, heroin, crack cocaine and OST – are feeling increasingly misunderstood and unwelcome at drug services. Drug policies and services, therefore, are intimately involved in how some bodies are made to matter over others, and it should be no surprise that it is for these people who use opiates and are no longer in treatment that the risk of death is greatest (ACMD, 2016; PHE, 2017). These failures to respond to these ways of doing drugs are a material issue of the most serious order. The second kind of movement getting mobilised does not rely so heavily on abstention and breaking habits as a detachment of the body from the substance, but, instead, on making new habits or rather *working within* habits to increase bodies' capacities to affect and be affected. This approach holds hope for a more 'hands-on' situated, specific and speculative intervention.

Movement as abstinence: breaking habits

An ontological politics is crucial to this account of movement as this is not so much about how service providers interpreted the recovery agenda – how it was known – but what was made in practice. That is, many participants embraced a more fluid account of recovery; however, this is not what always emerged. My intention, of course, is not to devalue what people told me, but more precisely to consider the forms of agency also occurring in less conscious and cognisant ways. I will look at the role policy, mutual aid groups and metaphor all play in habits that people are said to be 'stuck in', which rely on 'recovery' to 'unstick' them through, for example, group work and positive risk-taking. As such, 'the problem' of addiction and 'solution' of recovery seemed to coalesce around movement, mutually intra-acting in defining one another. Following Barad (2007), causes and effects are part of the same onto-epistemological apparatus. That is, here, addiction gets produced as breakable by the very technologies that try to break it – 'the solution' produces 'the problem'. This dynamic is particularly well highlighted in the case of methadone-reduction prescriptions, which were becoming the norm during my time at the Dunswell service, and in funding schemes, where services were not paid for those clients returning within six months (now increased to twelve months, Home Office, 2017). That is, an addiction to opiates, once seen as a relapsing condition, is reworked as something that can be rapidly weened and not returned to within a significant amount of time. Therefore, those service users who were less able to perform this latest version of addiction and its recovery by carrying out such detachments (breaking habits) were finding it harder to engage in support services.

Returning to the Dunswell service to carry out research in 2014, having volunteered there the previous year, from 2012 to 2013, I soon became aware of the changes the recovery agenda was having to what it meant to 'engage in treatment', where a stricter movement was intended, both through the service and in life towards becoming drug-free. As an explicit example, Narcotics Anonymous (NA), which works to a twelve-step, abstinence-based model, was getting suggested as a support service within the sector, and Public Health England representatives, with NA Fellows, came into the service to advocate for NA as part of a wider UK campaign (HM Government, 2015). The metaphor of 'stuck' played a key role in this construction of movement as abstinence. Following Fraser and valentine's (2008) idea that metaphors in drug environments are particularly powerful actants, the concept of being 'stuck' *does* something.

To offer some context, the word was commonly used to describe service users who found abstinence-based recovery difficult. In the interviews, it was also used by a regional director to describe parts of grass-roots harm reduction services that were considered no longer fit for purpose as he expressed a desire to 'get rid of the old and stuck'. When I was volunteering at the Dunswell service, two recovery workers were recruited to carry out cognitive behavioural therapy (CBT)-centred recovery-based sessions with clients that were described as 'stuck'. Interestingly, as previously stated, when I returned to the service a year later, all drug workers (called 'substance misuse practitioners') had been renamed 'recovery workers', thus, engaged in this 'unsticking' work. The 'stuck' metaphor came to my attention most acutely in a training session on neurolinguistic programming. This session focussed on these 'stuck clients' and looked at how workers could change clients' behaviours by shifting what were perceived to be their negative thought patterns through positive language to help them 'move forward'. Undoubtedly taking this on board, in my interview with Angela, she states: 'the recovery model thing is about *not being stuck in the reasons* of using, it's about thinking about your strengths'.

Recovery then becomes about 'unsticking', which included an increasing use of activities and group work. But, as Angela also asks: 'are we pushing people to do too much?'

FD: Like, is there more emphasis on trying to get people to engage in groups and that sort of thing rather than just coming for the script?

ANGELA: Yeah, definitely. So we've been told this over and over [by management]. There is an emphasis on more group work, more mutual aid, support groups, but there's also an emphasis on, there's also this thing at the moment where the government really want people, to push people into work, so when you get clients coming in or people who are coming in and then they're going to the job centre and they're being penalised if they don't attend the job centre and it's like, well, *are we pushing people to do too much?* [...] It just feels like we're living in a culture of things, *your life just constantly has to be taken up.*

Angela alludes to a tension in the ideals of recovery and the practical realities which enacts a state in which people can easily fail. But, as Angela points out, drug services should not be seen in isolation, rather part of what she calls a 'culture of things' in which 'your life just constantly has to be taken up', or controlled, including having to attend the job centre, but one could also assume social services, probation, housing services, as well as having family and other social responsibilities. It is such stifling environments that Peta Malins (2017) warns us about in a drug treatment sector that tries to inhibit rather than open up desire in what Deleuze and Guattari (1983) call a fascist 'control society'.

At the Eastford service, there had been an even more dramatic shift towards group work, in which one-to-one working had essentially ended. One worker, Karolina, says, with the caveat of being a cynic: 'I associate it with cutting down on costs, it's much cheaper to shove ten people into a group than to deliver one-to-one sessions'. Partly due to becoming disenchanted with these changes, Karolina had recently left the sector. She says:

> We had people storming out of the group and saying this is not for me, which was very embarrassing by the way because I was made to then call the client and offer one-to-one after the client was told that we don't offer one-to-ones.

It was only when the client became distressed and threatened to discharge themselves that their request for one-to-one work was granted.

Another treatment shift, which is perhaps in most stark opposition to a previous harm reduction ethos of the 1990s and 2000s, was a move to what might be considered positive risk-taking. Callum, the interim manager at the Dunswell service, notes how doctors' natural position of safety ('do no harm') is at odds with the need to take risks in recovery-focussed treatment. Talking about OST, I asked, 'do you think there is a bit of a conflict between the sort of medical prescribing model and the recovery model?', and he resolutely responded:

> There absolutely is. And it really is a *conflict between the risk management way of dealing with prescribing and the recovery means of dealing with prescribing.* If you use your prescribing to assist with recovery then you are going to have to at some point be taking a *risk.* I've had many practitioners say to me that I shouldn't be aiming to assist a client *becoming abstinent* because that would put the client at greater risk of overdose should they lapse and they're far safer if they remain on an opiate substitute script because then they're much less likely to overdose and die. This is obviously absolutely true, objectively, but then there's a person involved with *choices* and with a quality of life that needs to be supported and if that person wants to, you know, if we're saying to people we're not going to assist you to become abstinent then what are we doing here really.

Breaking habits involves taking risks, including the possibility of overdose, but, for Callum, this is a risk worth taking in re-covering the autonomous drug-free subject, that is, covering up our relationality in a 'control society' (Deleuze and Guattari, 1983) based on ideals of individual freedom. Worryingly, and taking this control further, Callum suggested that recovery-focussed prescribing might be better achieved when doctors are employed directly by the services (a model now commonly employed, including by the organisation who ran the Eastford service and in other services run by the Dunswell umbrella organisation).

However, as indicated in citing other workers' objections, this risk-taking had not gone unnoticed or uncriticised. Indeed, commentators have suggested a link between the recovery agenda and the recent dramatic rises in drug-related deaths (Woods, 2016). Heroin-related deaths increased by nearly two-thirds from 2012 to 2014 (during the fieldwork period) in England and Wales (ONS, 2015), and are currently at their highest levels on record (ONS, 2018). In a frank opinion piece in the popular UK drug service magazine *Drink and Drug News*, a service user group coordinator in London, Alex Boyt (2014), asks: 'Could the recovery agenda be killing people?' Boyt argues that by drug services taking a recovery focus, particularly through stricter methadone regimes, such as mandating additional group work, they could be alienating those not ready for abstinence:

> Many for whom recovery, especially in its abstinent form, is just too painful, difficult or unattractive. For this lot, often those most at risk from death and disease, the recovery agenda makes services less relevant and safe. People who used to be held by the treatment system are now confronted by goals for *integrating into society* the moment they make it through the door.
>
> (2014: 7, my emphasis)

As the recovery agenda produced addiction in a way that is 'breakable' (recover-able), some workers became increasingly frustrated with what to do with those clients that continued to use drugs and did not necessarily want recovery in these abstinence-based terms. During my time at the Dunswell service, a worker regularly vented his aggravations to me in relation to one service user in particular, Malik. Malik turned up most weeks feeling angry with himself having used 'on top' of his OST script. Speaking to Malik in the interviews for this project, he explained to me how he both wanted to use drugs and didn't want to – a contradiction that these strict forms of addiction and recovery (addiction-recovery) find difficult to handle. This resulted in a violent internalised conflict, which gets dramatically depicted in his body map (Figure 5.1).

Asked to describe the feelings after he uses drugs, Malik draws a picture of him shooting himself through the head, with a sign saying 'all sense gone this way', to indicate that, although he does not want to use drugs, there is something that still pulls him towards it. Interestingly, it is 'sense' that has lost out, which suggests, more than a fight against himself, this is a battle of sense over desire, or indeed, mind over matter. In considering this in relation to the stuck metaphor and the enactment of movement as an 'unsticking', especially through the use of cognitive and neurolinguistic techniques/therapies, recovery could be tightening a mind versus

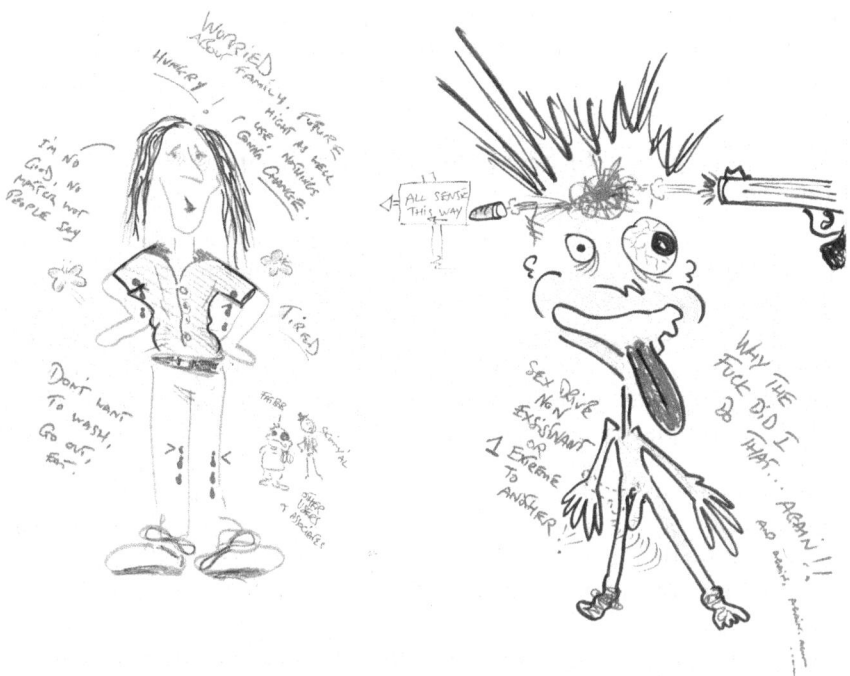

Figure 5.1 Malik's body map.

body conflict. This gets accentuated further in Malik's sentence, saying, 'why the fuck did I do that... again!!', writing 'And again, again, again' until there is no more space left on the paper. He is infuriated with himself for continuing to use drugs even though he does not want to. Addiction as recover-able and recovery as abstinence-focussed struggles to hold these two contradictory feelings together – wanting to and not wanting to use drugs – and, appears, in fact, to help play them off one another in positioning the mind – with choices – as capable of controlling the body. This is a key premise of cognitive-behaviour therapies recommended in recovery-based treatment (e.g. SMART recovery, n.d.).

Although Callum's views on recovery were not shared by all, they point to some of the more troublesome ways the recovery agenda was getting enacted in an abstinence-focussed way. That is, policy, metaphor, neurological knowledges, practitioners and funding strategies were intra-acting to produce restrictive forms of movement towards abstinence, which could inadvertently act to alienate some drug users from using services and contribute towards them internalising their desires as destructive conflicts – their movement (perhaps towards more careful, safer or reduced drug use) was not enough, not certain or controlled enough. I turn now to the specific place of methadone and reduction prescriptions as a key point of departure from previous harm reduction policies in this move towards recovery as abstinence.

'Breaking the power of prescribing': the case of methadone

Methadone prescribing has always been a contentious issue due to its substitutional (even supplementary) composition to illicit opiates such as heroin (Gomart, 2002a). But these debates have grown fiercer with the move to recovery-centred drug policy and services in the UK, but also overseas (Berridge, 2012; Duke et al., 2013; Lancaster et al., 2015). Indeed, in some governmental literature, the recovery agenda's key aim is precisely 'to shake up' methadone's place in heroin treatment (Home Office, 2012). Here, I want to gesture to the intra-action of media, film, policy and, again, metaphor, in the construction of methadone as a substance that holds such habit-forming potential or 'power' that it needs 'breaking'. This adds to Fraser and valentine's position that 'methadone is [best] not seen in terms of *a priori* attributes, rather as a phenomenon produced in specific intra-actions with other phenomena' (2008: 56).

Both service providers and users spoke of people being 'parked' and 'trapped' on methadone, which can be seen to plug into the 'stuck' metaphor and construction of recovery as movement. Angela, for example, says 'I mean some people have been stuck on a script for years'. The term and broader construct clearly reflects the enactment of methadone as a substance deeply entangled in discourse. The 'think tank', The Centre of Social Justice and its founder, Conservative politician, Iain Duncan Smith, have vehemently campaigned against methadone prescribing, which is said to 'replace one addiction for another', using the rhetoric of being 'parked' (used repeatedly in their documents). As such, they advocate for time-limited prescriptions and welfare benefit sanctions for those who 'use on top' or fail to comply (CSJ, 2013; 2014). Along these lines, buprenorphine is put forward as an alternative to methadone, claimed to produce more effective and quicker 'recovery' (through a 'rapid detox'), which fits with a notion of positive risk-taking noted above.

In terms of the popular media, perhaps one of the most prominent figures for his views on methadone is TV celebrity, Russell Brand. During the study period, he presented two BBC (2012; 2014) programmes on the issue, *From Addiction to Recovery* and *End the Drugs War*. Both portray a damning image of methadone as enslaving users, again using the metaphor of being 'parked'. Needless to say, his programmes have received widespread condemnation from drug activist groups (INPUD, 2015; SSDP, 2014). Popular culture, including film, has also participated in this negative enslaving imaginary, for instance, in the famous 1990s adaptation of *Trainspotting*,

Renton's mother, encouraging his attempt at 'cold turkey', says 'no methadone, you're worse on methadone'. A BBC Radio 4 (2016) programme, *Choose Life*, openly discusses this consciously taken stance. Within this changing environment, using an opiate substitute, such as methadone, and to a lesser extent buprenorphine, was becoming an increasingly unacceptable way to engage in services in the long term.

Therefore, in explaining how he recently restructured a neighbouring service, a structure which he was planning to import to the Dunswell service, Callum explicitly reflects on how he wanted to shift attention, both the workers' and service users' attention, away from prescribing and towards recovery:

> The engine of the service was prescribing…what we wanted to do in doing the restructure was, as it were, was to *break the power of prescribing* as the whole driver of everything that happened within the service and to create a situation where service users could have all the different recovery-based interventions that we had available open to them all the time so we wanted to move people's focus on to recovery away from prescribing.

The prescribing aspect of the service was seen to be limiting key-working conversations to what he and others called 'script talk' – discussing how the person is feeling on their methadone or buprenorphine prescription – rather than encouraging people to talk about and thereby focus their attention on recovery (moving towards abstinence).

> But what I do observe about this service [Dunswell] is that it is as [the restructured service] used to be, entirely driven by the scripting process. The fact that it's driven by the scripting process means that the conversation that is happening with the workers is less focused on care work, 'where do we go from here', 'where's the recovery?', 'when are you going to be coming off these drugs?', 'what's going on for you?', 'how do we move you forward?' and 'how do you feel this week, can we go down?' So my concern here is that we're not really having that discussion, we're telling ourselves that people aren't willing to *move on* because we're not giving them the time, and having the conversation.

Continuing to stress movement in this particular way, the future is then equated with abstinence in a way that to talk about the present is to limit this movement:

> And if you're always living in the present in terms of how you're doing now, rather than talking about the future, then of course you never have a conversation about reduction, and it would be quite easy for people to weasel out of that discussion if it comes up.

This stress on movement seems to be doing something else. Not only is there a focus on the future rather than the present, as if the two are mutually exclusive, but this movement towards abstinence is the only legitimate way of moving. So, for clients to talk about their OST is to 'weasel out' of this focus on an OST-free future. In a similar vein, observing a clinical training session with senior members of the organisation, we were told that we should be channelling service users' attention towards their drug use, and, if they brought up other issues like health, housing and employment, this could be a way of distracting us and themselves (linked to two concepts widely applied to addictive behaviours: manipulation and denial) from the 'real problem' – the drug use. That is, *moving* towards safer drug use or improving one's life in other ways was not enough.

This perhaps suggests a dramatic return to some of the attitudes prevalent in the pre-1990s, as explored in Emilie Gomart's (2002a; 2002b; 2004) famous work on France's first methadone programme. During this time, methadone was viewed to interrupt an ideal of freedom based on the autonomous subject:

> they held indeed that freedom can be measured by the autonomy of the agent's actions, that is, by the absence of exterior 'obstacles' to the implementation of an original intention or plan [...] A narcotic drug cannot be therapeutic, only destructive for the user.
>
> (2002a: 518–19)

Where Gomart observes methadone treatment to rework these ideals of freedom, enacting a *relative* freedom or 'generous constraint', I was conversely noticing a return to freedom based on autonomy (an 'absence of exterior "obstacles"'). Troubling 'recovery' is therefore about troubling what it means to be free.

Following the view that OST interferes with individual freedom, some service providers saw it as a form of 'collusion' (a common term in drug treatment contexts) to the point that services became seen as drug dealers: 'so I think services will be given less money to provide drugs to drug users' (Callum). In a similar light, Phil, who works for the drug service commissioning authority, says: 'you're just giving them another thing that ensnares and traps them in addiction'. This could de-legitimise people's claim to opiate substitution, making it harder for recipients to negotiate continued maintenance.

> It's a great millstone that people wear [weighing them down]. And it is a drug. It affects your consciousness, and you feel more dopey when you're taking methadone than when you don't. So you're not leading as clear and *fulfilling a life* as you possibly could be leading.
>
> (Callum)

From these standpoints, methadone and other opiate substitutes become part of the problem rather than the solution. Therefore, as Callum says, various steps are starting to be taken to break this power – a mystic quality that methadone is seen to have over its recipients as well as the service and its workers. During my time at the service, these steps included dividing the staff into prescribing and recovery teams, so prescribing could become more 'contractual' rather than 'therapeutic'; encouraging clients to 'work' for their scripts (e.g. by taking part in group activities); but most notably, and where I turn to next, reducing people's OST prescriptions. Indeed, continuing to talk with candid honesty, Callum suggested that everybody at the restructured service was now on a reduction prescription. 'Incidentally everybody in [that service] is on a reducing script. There isn't anybody who's on a maintenance script'. Surprised by this and enquiring further as to whether maintenance really isn't an option, Callum clarifies:

> It is in reality but everybody has a reduction plan, whether they stick to it or not is another matter. What you do get is a little bit of a roller coaster with some people, so they reduce a bit and then they say to the doctor that they're not feeling so good so the doctor increases it.

Although, again, it is hard to say how widespread these views and procedures are, they do reflect governmental goals (Home Office, 2010; 2017), especially those expressed in the document, Medications in Recovery: Re-Orientating Drug Dependence Treatment (NHS, 2012), and correspond to my observations and what participants told me about various services they attend in London. For example, one time at the Dunswell service, when I was asked to see a client for another worker who was on annual leave, the client was very pleased to see me. He explained with some trepidation that he had been on methadone for fifteen years, was 'stable', had a 'nice flat' and was not using illicit drugs (employing perhaps old markers for what 'successful' treatment may have looked like), but said that his worker had been asking him to reduce his methadone prescription (something that was regularly encouraged in the team meetings). The man must have been in his sixties and was resolute about not wanting to reduce his prescription this late on in his life. I reassured him (although I realise now this was perhaps misguided) that as far as I knew he did not have to reduce and we eventually agreed that he would continue this discussion with his key worker.

Anxieties around reductions were widely shared amongst participants, for example, Meg says:

> They're really, really, like this last year or so, they're really pressuring people to come down, cos I have come down, I was on about 75[mls] and I'm on 45 now, and they really are pressurising people to come off. I think it's all politics. If I'd just started and they offered some fast

treatment but when people have been on it for years, I think it's mad, just trying to rush them like that, they just want you to get down to 30ml, go to [detox] and just get off in two weeks, having been on it for twenty years, and they really seriously think that. People will just come out and buy brown [heroin] again. It just doesn't work, not that quick, it's too quick. I think 30mls in two weeks is ridiculous.

(Meg)

As Meg is pointing out here, a set of habits established over several years cannot be so easily broken. There was also often contention over coming off the last few millilitres. Service providers, perhaps with recourse to their neurolinguistic training on positive thinking, often felt that it was easier than recipients did.

They really are putting the pressure on people, but the thing is, coming down 5mls when you're on 70 is nothing but coming down 5mls when you're only on 20 is a big deal, cos the lower you get you really feel it [...] It is so hard, and you wouldn't think, cos you can drop 10mls when you're on 90 or something and you won't even notice it but the last 10mls you're in agony.

(Meg)

Also speaking on this issue, Silvie says:

I stopped for one year, [illicit] drugs, I was on methadone, but then I tried to cut down and I arrived at one point, and then it was very difficult [...] They [service providers] said it was psychological, *but it wasn't psychological*. The last 10/15mls was really difficult and I was really ill and I went to a Chinese [medicine] doctor and he said that you're putting your body through too much, you can't cut down that quickly, you have to be really careful, my body went into shock.

Silvie and Meg's narratives raise questions over time-limited methadone prescribing and the increasing advocacy for short-term buprenorphine, which could work to exclude those long-term users less willing or able to make such changes. As Silvie points out, methadone reduction was not a psychological issue, but a very real, material one – her 'body went into shock'. We need to start taking these habits seriously to avoid some of the unintentional harms, including the internalised conflicts as dramatically depicted in Malik's case, and those potentialised or afforded by services as they become less attractive to longer-term drug users who are often some of the most vulnerable people in society, with complex health needs. Additionally, as drug services shifted to a movement based on abstinence, not only was using opiate substitution for a long time becoming less acceptable, but so too was using illicit drugs 'on top' which, for example, in Gomart's time of writing, was once tolerated, even, as a method of stabilisation, endorsed.

'Using on top'

Where opiate substitution was once a legitimate way to reduce or 'stabilise' illicit drug use and all the associated harms, using both illicit drugs and licit OST (or 'using on top') was now actively discouraged. Increasingly, there seemed to be very little space for using OST in this way, which meant, for some participants, they had stopped picking up methadone altogether and preferred to buy it on the black market, which allowed a more flexible way of negotiating their drug use. This resonates with Harris and Rhodes's (2013a) analysis of methadone diversion as a protective strategy against biosocial harms, such as hepatitis C, in arguing for more flexible or 'generous' methadone programmes. I will suggest, in regard to stabilisation and maintenance, that such programmes were getting increasingly ungenerous, and producing potentially harmful forms of 'methadone subjects', 'addiction' and 'freedom'.

As seen above, methadone is becoming less acceptable, but, more specifically, it is becoming less acceptable as a harm reduction device for stabilising or reducing 'on top' use. In valentine's (2007) Australian study, she observes how the subject gets made with methadone as a 'stable user'. Methadone in this sense refigured ideas on addiction as something beyond the drug – 'methadone use can coincide with illicit drug use and, further, that illicit drug use does not erase the effects of methadone in addressing addiction' (valentine, 2007: 505). There was no longer the addict or non-addict, but variations in degree. In contrast, what I observe in the UK is a revival of the autonomous, free individual, where methadone too is part of the addiction ('the power').

Therefore, where valentine (2007) observes relatively polite, even positive co-constructions of subjects *with* methadone, such as 'the stable user, the individual in need of guidance, and the lay carer', I noticed more negative constructions. Such subjects included the 'messer'. The 'messer' describes somebody who uses illicit drugs, usually heroin, 'on top' of their prescription. Indeed, the fact that such use is called 'on top' already denotes the non-compliance of using licit and illicit substances together. Where 'messers' got identified in team meetings, the manager would remind workers to read them the terms of treatment, with the underlying assumption that they could be discharged if they failed to comply. Although this was often a threat more than a reality, it perhaps suggests where such policies might be heading. For example, the government recently explored the possibility of even sanctioning welfare benefits for those not complying to drug treatment, or, in other words, to OST regimes (Wintour, 2015).

There are, of course, legitimate reasons for services' concerns over 'on top' use as methadone is an opiate agonist and could contribute to an overdose. However, limiting one's concerns to this singular effect fails to take seriously the contingency of this effect and also some of the benefits found in mediating heroin consumption with methadone (Harris and Rhodes, 2013a). For some participants, methadone, or even buprenorphine in Dimitri's account in Chapter 3, was used to manage their illicit heroin use, and, as such, was sometimes not taken daily. Participants talked about wanting to avoid a 'double habit', which meant they sometimes preferred not to take their methadone. Gwen points out: 'you can't stop taking the heroin because you want to, and then you're taking both, so you've got a double habit, you've got a double habit, it's pointless'. Some participants, like Gwen, did not use drug services as a result, and others were careful to negotiate heroin use so not to miss their methadone dose (when they weren't using heroin) on three consecutive days which, according to clinical guidelines, meant they had to 're-start' treatment. With payment-by-results, such service uses (who find it harder to conform to these methadone regimes) may become a less attractive group to treat as they are seen to put treatment successes at risk – they are constructed as 'leaving' treatment with 'failed' treatment episodes. Again, talking frankly on how this 'cherry picking' might play out, Callum explains:

> So, using opiates and crack you've got about 4% potential likelihood of completing, if you're using opiates on their own, you've got maybe a 7% likelihood of completing. Whereas if you're a cannabis user you've got a 40% likelihood of completing or powder cocaine user, you've got a 40/35% chance of completing, whereas if you were a crack only user, you've got maybe a 30% chance. [The problem with the Dunswell service] is that *they are not targeting anybody other than opiate users* so of course we have those completion rates because those are the completion rates you get for opiate users

FD: Right, so getting different sorts of drug users then, it's likely to increase the completion rates?

> Yes, so one of the things I'm trying to do here now is offer services to a wider range of drug users because I know that I'll get better completions for those drug users and that will bring the average for [the Dunswell service] to a state that is more comparable than other boroughs cos in other boroughs they're offering a more holistic service for people using a range of things. And you will have seen it here everybody at [the Dunswell service] is an opiate user.

Therefore, not only are people on long-term (maintenance) opiate prescriptions becoming less attractive to treat, and those using illicit opiates 'on top', but so are those using opiates more generally, trying to access treatment.

Furthermore, new outcome measures stipulate that the treatment completion was no longer 'successful' if the service user returned within a six-month period. This curiously enacts addiction in a different way to the dominant neurological models that define it as a 'chronic relapsing condition' (NIDA, 2015; see also Lancaster et al., 2015). Instead, it is enacted as recover-able. Speaking on this point, Dr Green says that drug addiction is no longer seen as a relapsing condition in treatment provision as clients have to focus on long-term recovery and funding will be lost if people relapse.

FD: Is drug use still seen as a chronic relapsing…?

DR GREEN: No, no, I don't think, *I think there is so much emphasis on long term recovery*, and I think for instance if you close someone as treatment completed but they come back within six months, you soon will lose your funding and will lose your credit for that previous successful completion because they are coming back into treatment. So, one of the commissioners will say well that wasn't successful, because they came back, which is interesting, cos in a way for us we want people to come back as soon as possible when they are at risk of relapse and start supporting them again… If somebody, you know, does become drug free and relapses I want them to feel comfortable to come back to treatment as soon as possible, whereas targets that say, you know, if they re-present in a certain number of months *aren't conducive to services being welcoming back of those people* because they know that those people will make their targets worse. And yet relapses are a common part of addiction and so it seems to me like some of those targets are potentially counter-productive and you know can discourage good care.

As well as producing a different kind of addiction as breakable, Dr Green points to the potential risk such regulations pose to 'good care'. Such models, as we have already seen, could lead to 'cherry picking'. For example, Nyundo, the manager at the Eastford service, comments:

I think if you miss out on harm reduction you end up *cherry picking* who you work with, because people are in different places in recovery and their drug use and some people, as much as people want to brag about our models and our great services, some people are going to use drugs and there's nothing you can do about it, and it's their choice in a way.

Although these more complicated views of addiction were widely shared amongst service providers, certain technologies, such as the outcome measures (pressing for faster completion rates), worked against them. The needle exchange facility at the Eastford service also now took a recovery focus. Nyundo says: 'you can get people coming into the needle exchange and talk to them about what their next steps are and publicise and market the services that you have for recovery'. Therefore, although, in theory, space was carved out for both clients engaging in abstinence-based recovery and harm reduction, in practice, often it was recovery that dominated. The concern here is that those wanting to continue using illicit drugs will feel less inclined to come to the facilities where the expertise is on hand. Indeed, the vast majority of participants in this study accessed needles over-the-counter at pharmacies, for, rather conversely, if the drug service knew they were using drugs, it could jeopardise their treatment and opiate prescription, especially if they take it home, as they were supposed to be abstinent from illicit substances to qualify.

To conclude this section on breaking habits, we can see how a specific kind of addiction and movement towards abstinence is taking hold, which arguably works against the routines and practices entangled in the lives of many people (in the making) who inject drugs. The less generous methadone strategies become, the more harmful these forms of methadone subjectivity ('messer'), addiction (as breakable) and freedom (outside of treatment structures and support services) also become. However, at the same time as some of these narrow enactments of recovery were taking place, there were also more flexible ones, which could take habits more seriously. If we understand habits as the sociomaterial practices that modulate our capacities to affect and become affected, then we are always living through habits. Therefore, moving from attachment (being stuck, parked) to detachment (individual freedom, 'unsticking') makes little sense. Where recovery is based on a premise of addiction as breakable and the individual's autonomy as restorable, and harm reduction is based on the individual's autonomy and rights as preordained and insurmountable, then where I want to go next is to explore the potential of those care practices in the drug services that were based on *relationality*. Service providers worked within constraints and most notably *with* habits in a set of practices I call more-than-harm reduction. Instead of focussing on the drug, and trying to make people detach from drugs, some practitioners talked of working within this relationality, in making new habits, whether this included drugs or not.

More-than-harm reduction: working with habits

Where I have drawn attention to some of the limiting ways the recovery agenda was getting made in the services to the exclusion of some people (given that people are made with/through habits), this section draws attention to some of the parallel ways recovery was also enacted in a more inclusive way. Unlike the previous section which presented an approach to recovery as a way of ending habits based on a substance and a set of breakable connections – the body from the drug – this section looks at how recovery was also occurring in a way that was more sensitive to the various capacities in which we are all machined by our habits. This may present a way of engaging with recovery discourses (prevalent in today's global drug

policies) in less exclusionary and harmful ways. Working with habits enacts a more intimate form of caring for injecting bodies on their own terms
(as they make themselves known) in what one participant called 'harm reduction and *more*' (to emphasise the production/movement). That is, some
service providers neither identified as working within a recovery *or* harm
reduction frame, but rather between the two, in more-than-harm reduction.
This was about more than reducing harm, but less than a strict recovery
dependent on abstinence. First, I will attend to how these practices focussed
on habits beyond the drug. Second, I will look at how they take place within
constraints and disrupted these traditional treatment divides.

During my time at the Dunswell service, a new 'strengths based' assessment tool was introduced to gather information on people wanting to start
treatment. This tried to turn the focus away from the drug use as the perceived problem towards a more general focus on things that were going well
in people's lives. Where the previous assessment form asked 'reasons for
drug use', this one did not. It was even quite far down the list of questions
that it asked anything about drugs. Angela reflects on this shift:

> I think what the 'strength based' model and the recovery model thing
> is about is not about being *stuck* in the reasons of using [drugs and al-
> cohol], it's about thinking about your strengths and not [cuts herself
> off] ... So, what you find with new workers that come in now is that they
> have this real kind of positive attitude about *not being a drug user* rather
> than working with *you are a drug user*. And things have got you here and
> let's think about that to try and *unfold stuff, so that it doesn't continually
> repeat itself.*
>
> (Angela)

This is a very different approach to the 12-step idea, which pins people to
the addict identity, that is, once an addict always an addict. For Angela,
drug use is just one part of her clients' lives and to focus on something other
than the drugs is a way to *make new habits*. Rather than focussing on the
drug (as promoted in the clinical training session) to change or break habits, the focus is on the other aspects of clients' lives, so that new habits will
change old ones. Angela also uses the language of folds, which speaks to a
folding of outer and inner worlds, and the constant entanglement of the two
in modulating participants' capacities to act.

Furthermore, moving recovery away from the drug habit per se to a wider
idea of making new habits, the manager at the Eastford service, Nyundo,
was very keen for the service to become *more than a drug service* and had
recently designed a 'recovery café' to be situated in the service's kitchen.

> We're opening up a recovery café, so people can come and have a nice
> safe space to socialise in. I think in general a lot of what we are trying to

do is break down the walls to treatment and *open up a bigger experience* for people so they can have a bit more life, a bit more activities that are *not just treatment,* so in the programme we talk about your relationship with yourself, your relationship with the world, we think about citizenship, we think about social justice, so it's just a very interesting way to start thinking about drug treatment, and really trying to address people quite holistically.

This approach is about expanding ideas of recovery beyond abstention, to develop other parts of people's lives.

There is a genuine curiosity and modesty to the approach that seeks to allow service users, in their fullness (relationality), to define what is best for them. Workers wanted to know the clients in their full event-fullness, made up of their environments, social relationships, housing, jobs and the many roles these engender – rather than seeing them as a 'drug user' or just another 'number', as Angela used to often retort in team meetings. By seeking to mediate rather than remove attachments, working with habits is a care practice that appreciates the routines and positive effects that drugs can produce. For instance, Eva, a recovery worker at the Dunswell service, says 'I think the prescribing kind of works for the physical dependency but it does not work for the addiction to the ritual, so some people will just continue injecting'. And Karolina, who was until recently a recovery worker at the Eastford service, points to a need for less structure and more *genuine curiosity*:

> So, I would actually express *genuine kind of curiosity* about the pleasure and what they are enjoying, not because it's a treatment strategy or because I'm supposed to do it, *but because it helps me to understand the person more.*

Nyundo also reflects on how this mode of care affords inclusion and openness to difference in how drugs get experienced:

> ...for a lot of people it will alleviate boredom, for a lot of people it'll help their mental health, for a lot of people it'll be a great way to socialise, so you really have to work with that because that's the things they want to explore with you, and think about how can you socialise, how can you enjoy yourself, how can you get a bit of a kick out of life, for instance, a lot of the newer drugs, it's very much about sex, how can you have a good sex life without it. If you forget about that and just focus on why shouldn't you use this, why is this bad for you, why are you going to put yourself at risk and pickup sexually transmitted diseases. If that's your first emphasis, well ultimately you're going to lose people.

We need to tap into these desires, for living well, rather than focussing on how to contain them.

Taking up a Deleuzian philosophy to living well, to fully potentialise one's power to act, Malins (2017) proposes an alternative treatment model based on desire (see also Duff, 2014a).

> Developing treatment approaches based on desire might [...] shift the focus away from stopping people taking drugs, to instead connecting them to new assemblages, such that they might continue to plug into desire flows, albeit through assemblages that might be healthier for them.
>
> (2017: 131)

Dr Green speaks to what such 'connecting' may look like and comments explicitly on the ways such an approach breaks down the harm reduction and recovery distinction.

> To my mind, the best of both worlds would be offering all those things about moving your life on-housing, support about housing, employment and education and all those things-alongside maintenance, where appropriate. Not to say that it's appropriate for everybody, some people are sure to have more resilience and perhaps more family support, more things that mean that a short treatment course is more appropriate, or you know a detox and short rehab and then move out of the drug treatment system. But I think that for many people who use drugs and alcohol have been *part of their life for a long time...* then often both are needed in parallel.

Dr Green recognises how bodies as movement are machined by 'things' – 'those things about moving your life on' – and therefore it is within this relationality that new bodies can emerge. This takes seriously not only our relationality, but the differences in how these 'things' are experienced and how certain detachments/attachments can be harder for some than others.

> And I see, personally, no problem, if somebody is doing well on maintenance, why that's a problem anymore than somebody being on medication for diabetes say. You still want a diabetic to lose weight and do exercise and eat healthy, but it's not to say you're pressuring the diabetic to stop taking medication, whereas, using that analogy with substance misuse, it sort of feels like, ok, now you should move on, whereas some people can be abstinent and function well and work on a maintenance prescription, but not do terribly well when they try and come off that. To my mind, from what I'm aware of in terms of the clinical evidence.

Where Dr Green's diabetic patients can have both long-term medication *and* lifestyle interventions, his drug-using ones cannot, even though, as he says, people 'function well and work on a maintenance prescription'. Through this comparison, drug 'misuse' is highlighted as a politically charged condition in which 'the evidence' is not prioritised.

Although there are increasing difficulties to practising what Dr Green calls the 'best of both worlds', some service providers continue to carve out territories for engaging between narrowly defined models of harm reduction and recovery. Workers perform the typical harm reduction work, but they also do more, in working with others, human and non-human, in creating new habits and ways of becoming-other. Therefore, it is not that the recovery and harm reduction are separate, indeed, for some, as one regional service manager insists, the separation has never existed, but that harm reduction can now do *more*.

Workers draw attention to the potentiality of life: 'it's having that thought that everyone has the potential to flourish and grow and develop'. Continuing, Angela says:

> Since having this recovery model with the harm reduction work, I've noticed that people's qualities of lives are really improving, not, maybe not for some in major ways, but for others, *just in small ways*, and they're really benefitting from getting up and going to work or maybe starting to volunteer, you know.

It is through these small gestures that new ways of becoming are made possible. Angela says: 'it's a bit like happiness or *a different way of being* then becomes their drug'. This resonates with Bennett et al.'s observation that 'habits, as parts of mind–body–environmental assemblages, and in which questions of dis- and rehabituation, are no longer posed as matters of changing the subject but as ones of modifying the arrangement of such assemblages' (2013: 12). These care practices are not about focussing on the individual, who is encouraged to become drug-free, but rather on the entanglements that must be collectively moved or worked with in ways to produce good affects and reduce bad affects.

Working more broadly within these networks, the drug becomes less important. It is about engaging *with* these connections rather than trying to recover a past autonomy. Most notably, it no longer matters so much if the person continues to take drugs or not.

> There's a balance of not putting too much pressure on people and kind of allowing people to really go at their own rate. Like, what I would say in a session is 'I'm here to see you whether you are on methadone, not on methadone, whether you smoke heroin, whether you don't smoke heroin, that's not my choice, I will see you each week, every fortnight, regardless, but what I am here to do is to kind of help to encourage the kind of things you want out of life'.
>
> (Angela)

Recovery, defined in this way, embraces a more fluid notion of movement. For Angela, there needs to be less of a focus on the drug as an entity with a causal effect (a position supported throughout this book), and more attention on the other relationships that make up people's lives. We are intra-relational beings and, therefore, drug use is just one aspect of our assembling bodies and capacities to act.

> If we don't sort out their housing we're never going to get them to that point where they're able to hold down some sort of long-term job, if we don't sort out what their immediate crises are, you know. If the family situation or those family connections aren't good [...] if we don't work on ways of trying to resolve those, then we're not going to get them to that end point.
>
> (Angela)

However, as seen above, drug workers are restricted too in what they can do. They spoke of a lack of resources, tensions between staff and management, along with restrictive policies, outcome measures and negative media images and metaphors that made this client work more challenging to work with than, say, those with diabetes. Service providers worked within these collectives to negotiate these restrictive forms to find more open ways of engaging in recovery beyond abstinence. This included 'fiddling with' (not separate from but in connection to) OST reduction plans, the needle exchange, time-limited interventions and outcome measures.

Talking about reducing OST doses, Angela says:

> But it's about doing it *gradual,* I know there's a lot of emphasis on numbers in treatment and all the rest of it but *I'd just go at my clients pace* and I wouldn't do it any quicker

For Nyundo, this ethos extends to the need for 'open access services', like the needle exchange, and building up relationships over time:

> I think that's where things like open access services are really important because that's where the person who needs a needle exchange will walk in and start to know people, unlock, almost – it is a difficult thing. And, quite often, with new people that's where we leave it, and then build up a relationship over time.

Karolina also expresses frustration with quick interventions and their inadequacy caring for those who require longer-term support, for habits that, as Nadiya in the epigraph says, 'have been a long time in the making'. Karolina explains how she had to be creative and 'fiddle' with those technologies that require rapid/fixed movement:

> It should always be in 12 weeks, but that's like the theory, that never worked for me. I was one of those worst offenders of keeping people in

treatment for a very long time [...] I almost feel guilt for holding people in treatment, like, *intuitively* you know that you can't discharge this person because they need support, then you've got your manager saying, you know, and quite rightly so, if you have this client, you can't see somebody else, you're getting funded to see somebody new [...] *It's really, really complicated.* It should be 12 weeks, but the most of the time it is not, you will have people that drop out and you will have people that only want counselling [...] There are people that have been on the case load for a long period of time and then you kind of *fiddle with it,* we do it, and [another drug service] do it as well, I know that one of the workers was sitting in a review meeting with social services and she said I have to close the case now but I'll re-open it next week. So, you have to be so *creative.*

Karolina worked collaboratively within these treatment collectives to disrupt fixed measurement outcomes. Rather than working objectively, from abstract goals, she employs her subjectivity and body (what she calls 'intuition') to 'creatively' overcome restrictions and support people in different ways, where some people want to stay for a long time and others just want counselling.

Karolina and Angela's practices are reminiscent of what science studies scholars have called 'tinkering' (Law, 2011; Mol, 2008; Moriera, 2010). For Annemarie Mol and colleagues (2010), tinkering is a mode of care which takes the technological, social and natural together, instead of the practitioner or patient having to take control.

For rather than insisting on cognitive operations, they involve embodied practices. Rather than requiring impartial judgements and firm decisions, they demand attuned attentiveness and adaptive tinkering.

(2010: 15)

Resisting these outcome measures did not necessarily mean abandoning them, but collaboratively working *with* them and others, such as the manager, funding schemes, outcome measures and service users (those 'dropping out' or 'needing more time') in negotiating care paths. She says how 'it's really, really complicated'. But instead of trying to gain control over this complexity, she works in mediation with these relations, or what Moreira (2010), in his study in a dementia care home, calls 'life collectives' for making things work. From this position, 'good care' is about 'persistent tinkering in a world full of complex ambivalence and shifting tensions' (Mol et al., 2010: 14).

In a similar way to Karolina, Simone, from the Dunswell service, explains how restrictive forms are negotiated. She recounts situations where clients have stopped using heroin, but wish to continue using crack every so often and therefore cannot be closed in any 'planned way':

> So, because we've had situations where some people say I just wanted to deal with my heroin, you know. I've come in, I've stopped heroin, but I still want to use crack once a week. And we can't close them in a planned way, because they're still using crack once a week.

She spoke about how there had been a change to the outcome measures or 'data sets', which meant there were now only two ways to record a 'successful completion', either they had to be 'drug-free' or an 'occasional user', but the category specified 'no heroin or crack'. She says: 'you could grade people in so many different ways, but then they took all those options away'. She therefore says how she has to close her ears when clients say they may continue using crack in order to recognise these client-defined successes, which would otherwise be recorded as treatment failures. Even though the measures dictated absolutes, workers tried to make them more flexible. Therefore, as Karolina summarises, it was often flexibility that was felt to be the key to good care:

> I think it's the one size fits all which is the actual problem. I don't think [group work] is a problem, I don't think the recovery agenda is a problem. I don't even think the funding is that much of a problem, if you ask me. I think it's this kind of thought that this one thing will work for everyone.

Consequently, in this third section of the chapter, I hope to have shown that where restrictive forms of recovery were taking place so too were more open forms. With some actants clearly overlapping (featuring in both sections), I am not trying to set up oppositional modes of treatment, but rather show how different entanglements (e.g. of outcome measures, assessment tools, policies, metaphors) come to produce different treatment constructs and subjects (e.g. of recovery, addiction, movement, freedom). For example, the strength-based assessment tools helped produce a focus on mind over matter in recovering individual choice, but, in sensitising workers to social and emotional growth, they also produced a recovery attentive to desire and becoming-other. It is through plugging into these latter forms that I argue below and in the concluding chapter that we can start to take drugged relationalities more seriously and work with habits to create better ways of becoming-with drugs.

Conclusion

> There [is] a lot of conflict between 'what is recovery?' and 'what is abstinence?' and you know, should we expect abstinence from people, should

we not, should we dictate to people what treatment is [...] How do you work with someone who has made the choice that they want to stay using drugs and injecting drugs and they're happy with that – how do you deal with that in a recovery model?

(Nyundo, manager, Eastford service)

There seems to be an enduring tension in drug treatment at the moment between more open and narrow discourses of recovery and how different ways of using drugs fit within them (or not). One seems to be producing more restrictive forms based on breaking habits, whilst another focusses more on changing habits, and intervenes (or 'tinkers') within these sociotechnical collectives. The latter, I argue, blurs the traditional divisions between harm reduction and recovery in producing *more than harm reduction*, based on movement and growth, whilst not being restricted by a movement towards abstinence. Therefore, as a tentative, yet serious, response to Nyundo's slightly rhetorical question, this wider onto-epistemology of movement and way of tinkering within habits (inhabited by drug users and service providers) may offer a way of practicing care beyond reductionist enactments of movement and its potential exclusions whilst remaining relevant in an era of recovery (hooked on movement) that looks like it's here to stay.

In understanding habit as affect modulation and thus part of our embodied capacity for change, not every*body* has the capacity (where capacity originates from one's sociomaterial make-up) for abstinence. This is not about an internal incapacity or lack, located in the body or psyche, but rather a displaced capacity located in flows of desire, making some people more able to make these changes than others. Russell Brand brings this to our attention when, in his programmes (cited above), he tries to transport what worked in his own recovery onto others, and, in particular, two women, who were experiencing extreme forms of marginalisation. It made extremely painful viewing as we watched them 'fail' at rehabilitation. It is vital that people are not pressurised or made to feel guilty for 'failing' to gain abstinence which is unequally available. That is, we need to have more understanding of our post-humanity in order to achieve a more compassionate, caring and, in many ways, more-than humane approach to drugs. As Matt puts it:

Not everybody wants abstinence. And I think that we have to understand that. The recovery agenda is fine but [...] *it is a fact that not everyone wants abstinence,* there are some people that just don't want to stop using but they don't want to use in such a way that they are going to kill themselves or they're going to have to do things that they consider are going to impact seriously on the quality of their lives.

By embracing a Deleuzian philosophy, we can think about health, following Duff (2014a), as 'the affective and relational force that impels a body's developmental trajectory, giving rise to the acquisition of novel competencies and thereby extending a body's scope of activity' (Duff, 2014a, 75). Thus, more emphasis is needed on how we come to be affected *and affect* (our capacity to become-other) – 'where we might be able to go and what we might be able to do' (Massumi, 2015: 3). This is not about being ruled by habits, but rather being made up of them:

> We have to be careful. If we say, 'I contract habits and then habits rule me', or 'We can remobilize habit for futurity', we are positing a subject, us or me, prior to and separate from the process of event-formation that habit is so central to.
>
> (Massumi, 2015: 65)

Employing a concept of habit as machinic, I have tried to trouble a very troubling enactment of recovery based on a set of breakable habits (with assumed separations between a subject and object, mind and body, individual and environment), which, as I argue, works to exclude some people (made up/through habits) more than others. In particular, this may be negatively affecting opiate users accessing treatment, long-term users of opiate substitution, especially methadone, and those who 'use on top'. However, where some workers seemed to be engaging in an alternative movement, they offer hope for alternative ways of working with recovery-based policies, whilst pushing against its more constraining and harmful potentials. In bringing the book to a close in the next and final chapter, I will look further at some of these openings for future intervention.

Conclusion

Empowering bodies: making bodies better?

In this concluding chapter, I consider in more detail a notion of power as the capacity to act gained from one's relationality and, therefore, the potential role for all of us in reconfiguring drug-using bodies in better, more empowered ways. Empowerment is a frequent term employed in drug-service provision and wider models of social care. Here, however, it takes on a distinctly more-than-human meaning. As we have seen, bodies are defined by their capacity to affect and be affected in their relational make-up. Disempowerment occurs where these potentials are reduced or 'blocked', whilst empowerment occurs where these are enhanced. By mapping injecting bodies, I hope to have shown where these points of empowerment and disempowerment can happen in participants' drug-using and -treatment practices to think, do and intervene-with drugs differently. Attending to this assemblic make-up of bodies, I argue that we can help enact injecting and drug-using bodies as a 'matter of care' (Puig de la Bellacasa, 2017). To develop this argument, I will first revisit a notion of empowerment as an embodied and ethico-political state. I will then look at where this empowerment could be harnessed and 'machined' in future drug research, treatment and policy as care work.

(Dis)empowerment is an embodied (in)capacity to act which cannot be disconnected from its assemblic formation. The social (political, economic, conceptual) and material context or situation fundamentally *matters*. As seen in Chapter 4 (to be discussed further below), it was not the drugs that meant participants went 'deeper and deeper into it' (addiction), but the 'way of life' – the lack of housing and support. Similarly, it was not only the chemical reaction of the drug with the neurotransmitters and respiratory system that meant participants nearly died of an overdose, but the illegality of the substance, which meant those around at the time were too fearful to call an ambulance. Or, for participants in Chapter 3, to feel a rush-relief from injecting, a number of *things* and techniques had to be in place. (Dis)empowerment is thus contingent on how power is eventualised in bodies' coming together and not simply a matter of causal effect (the drug chemically reacting with 'the body'), or, for that matter, individual choice.

We have seen in this book how drugs, commonly conceptualised as addictive, pathological or hedonistic, and thus confining of how some*body* can use and be on them, can actually help bodies, productively, to move, feel, act and think. Indeed, in Chapter 4, heroin (illegal and legal) became a fundamental part of participants' 'normal' or 'healthy' state. But such 'power' is specific to these contexts and thus we must pay attention to how it comes into being and emanates. Power is always a 'power to' rather than 'power from' – a power or freedom to act rather than a power or freedom from oppressive structures or, for this project, crucially, drugs. By understanding power as a positive force of life and the body as an enactment of this empowerment, defined by its assemblic make-up, we all become implicated in how bodies are done and could be done better, or in other words empowered, as an ethical and material imperative. It is with this that I return to the two framing questions of the book, stated in Chapter 1: How do we *do* injecting bodies? And how can we *do* them better?

I have argued that by becoming-with injecting bodies (described in Chapter 1), that is, by paying attention to their tensions (Chapter 2), attachments (Chapter 3), desires (Chapter 4) and habits (Chapter 5), we can potentialise different ways of thinking, practicing, living and intervening-with bodies. With this, I have shown how: pleasure can be considered in places where it might not have been otherwise; drug effects, more generally, are contingent; 'blockages' (or disempowerments) are relational and thus can be 'freed up' relationally; and habits, always in process, have to be re-made rather than un-made. Whilst I have tried to articulate these moments of empowerment throughout, I now attempt to explicate them further as an ethico-politics for making bodies better.

Here, I will hone-in and activate those already established more-than-harm reduction practices for making bodies better operating in people who inject drugs' own practices and at the two drug services. These were not dependent on making bodies free from drugs or injecting, but more loosely based on increasing their power to act, or what I now see as a collaborative effort to *make bodies better*. However, this is not about making them better from a distance – built on a normative idea of health, through a series of carefully measured and tested interventions. Instead, they were made better in participants' connections *with* such bodies – substances, paraphernalia, policy, concepts, biotechnologies, etc. Taking up Maria Puig de la Bellacasa's triptych of care as a vital doing, affective state and ethico-political obligation, this is a 'hands-on' process of *mattering*, in its double meaning as an ethical and political (to matter) and material (of matter) practice. Next then, in these concluding sections, I explore what this collective care (as doing-affect-ethics) may look like in future drug *research*, *treatment* and *policy*.

Speculative drug research

> Even more than before, knowledge as relating [...] matters in the mat-
> tering of the world.
>
> Maria Puig de la Bellacasa, 2017: 28

For some time now, critical drug studies have not only sought to better know or critique our current alcohol and other drug (AOD) ontologies and epistemologies, but get involved in these enactments. Therefore, I advocate for an approach that not only 'gets involved' (Law and Urry, 2004), but 'speculates' to create better worlds. Speculating, in Alex Wilkie, Martin Savransky and Marsha Rosengarten's (2017) edited collection *Speculative Research*, 'demands the active taking of risks that enable an exploration of the plurality of the present, one that provides resources for resistance, out of which unexpected events may erupt, and alternative futures may be created' (Savransky et al., 2017). Speculative research, conceived this way, is reliant on a topological understanding of temporality, like that seen in the third and last chapters, so that the future does not follow an arrow of time, but, like a handkerchief, is dependent on how it is 'spread, crumpled and torn' (Savransky et al., 2017). This is a kind of temporality that research does not merely add to in producing futures that learn from the present, but actually helps redesign – 'to pay attention to, and experiment with, the very *processes* of crumpling, folding and "tearing" time, and not just to their culmination' (Savransky et al., 2017). To be intimately entangled in this way in the AOD worlds we study requires a different mode of knowing based on our relationality, articulated here as becoming-with. And it is in rendering drug research in this way that 'touch', I argue, offers an alternative onto-epistemology to sight and sound for mattering the world speculatively, for 'cutting' worlds and bodies in different, 'better' ways.

By setting out an approach to injecting drug use based on bodies rather than subjects and their objects, I hope to have gone some way to establishing an alternative strategy for studying/knowing how drugs act and where to intervene in these more-than-human worlds. Considering research as a 'hands-on' practice of maintaining worlds, as a care practice, touch is a mode of simultaneously knowing and intervening in these worlds – as Puig de la Bellacasa (2017) and Barad (2007; 2012) point out – to touch is to be touched back. Unlike seeing and hearing, one cannot touch and not be touched back – 'this puts the question of reciprocity at the heart of thinking and living with care' (Puig de la Bellacasa, 2017: 20). Here, I think of drug-using and injecting bodies in these terms, to extend out their boundaries so we can become more accountable for their becoming.

Research performs 'agential cuts', that is, some things get included and others excluded (Barad, 2007). But this is not about a consciously chosen act of the author, rather, cuts are intra-actions of a sociomaterial making.

Divides and separations are something that get performed in the research assemblage. And, it is my assertion, following both Barad and Puig de la Bellacasa, via Haraway (1997; 2008), that with more 'response-able' methods and sensibilities we can make cuts that afford new relationships and connections. That is, the inevitable exclusions we make, if done response-ably, can engender bodily boundary-making that fosters empowerment rather than disempowerment. For example, seeing participants' becoming-with drugs as habit (Chapter 5) performs very different cuts to those seen in addiction discourses (like those seen in Chapter 1). Habits allow those social and material actors into our very embodiment that addiction holds outside as 'triggers'. Similarly, viewing pleasure as an embodiment of the assemblage is very different from seeing it as a causal effect of the drug-body interaction. And, by considering 'harms' and 'blockages' as the work of the 'slipping' injecting assemblage (Chapter 3) or stratification (Chapter 4), can hold us all to account in our interventions with people who use drugs. By paying attention to injecting and drug-using bodies, and becoming response-able to them, we can help to do them otherwise. That is, whilst we cannot care for everything, these cuts need not be seen to cut-off worlds (Puig de la Bellacasa, 2017), rather, new cuts, via our sensitised research practices, can foster new kinds of relationality and life.

Instead of following the usual dichotomies that split bodies, this book has tried to follow all sorts of bodies, human and not, that resist and struggle against such boundaries; blurring *a priori* divides between injecting equipment, people who inject, drug dealers, substances, policy documents, institutions, concepts, etc. Instead of cutting bodies down fixed lines, the research assemblage allowed bodies to flow, overspill and move between and beyond each other, to form new boundaries. Far from dumb, bodies have proven clever, responsive and even thinking. They moved each other in desiring and pursuing drugs; worked together to alleviate tolerance; pre-empted injecting events by going into withdrawals which could even heighten the high to come; collectively lost control in acts of pleasure; became habituated together; and gave up these habits by making other connections. We need new methods that can deal with these many ways that bodies can become-with drugs to nurture their possibilities for empowerment.

Making these different ways of becoming *matter* is not only an empirical pursuit but an ethical one, what Barad (2007) calls an 'ethics of mattering'. Not only can drug research produce new ways of knowing where 'the human subject is not the locus' (Barad, 2007: 393), but also the things known and made knowable. Therefore, where these realities are done in less careful ways – what we have seen in the tensions between pleasure and addiction (Chapter 2), the painful slippages in the injecting assemblage (Chapter 3), the blockages in becoming-other (Chapter 4) and failures to register certain kinds of bodies-as-movement (Chapter 5) – through our response-ability, we can help to enact them in more care-full ways: to think pleasure and addiction together; achieve pleasure in the injecting event; live bodies *with* drugs; and intervene-with habits. Having explored how touch and becoming-with re-invigorates our boundary-making as both a lively practice and one that we are all a part of, what does this mean for future research invested in making injecting and drug-using bodies better?

For this speculative effort, invention and creativity are key to open up possibilities otherwise closed down by our methods and disciplinary divides that privilege certain ways of using and 'treating' drugs, for example, as recreational or addictive, mental or physical, harmful or joyful. The body mapping method presented here has been pivotal in moving beyond the normative drug user and their body, but I now wonder what more could be done to further these disruptions. Speculative drug research should curate new relations of bodies, forces and things in a way that can allow for the differences in how drugs are done (that do not rely on predefined states), to do them in new and better ways. As I said above, research is about more than enacting realities (Law and Urry, 2004), but caring for them, or at least caring for some more than others. As researchers, involved in these processes, we become part of 'mattering the world' and, in this, response-able. *'Each of "us" is constituted in response-ability. Each of "us" is constituted as responsible for the other, as the other'* (Barad, 2012: 215, original emphasis). With such reciprocity, we are obligated to bring into being better ways of living with drugs in our more-than-human worlds.

Inevitably, this observation may leave the reader with more questions than answers. If we are to embrace our methodological role as researcher-creators, how might we begin to judge our interventions? That is, if the purpose of speculative research is to put at risk our research subjects, objects and relations as we know them, then how do we ensure they are known better? In our methods' capacities to *do* the social, they are also undoing the social – an assembling somewhere is always a disassembling somewhere else – and thus care, attention and reflexivity are needed. But, then, how do we acknowledge our role in these constructions without thinking this is all there is; how do we acknowledge that we are part of something bigger without returning to the 'crisis of representation' and self-reflexivity as an all-too-easy escape route? In Barad's terms, how do we take stock and stay critically aware of a world that will inevitably 'kick back'?

Situational drug treatment

More-than-harm reduction practices, as outlined in the previous chapter, refocus harm reduction towards both increasing good affects and reducing the bad. Indeed, these affects work in tight dynamism, for practices plugging into more positive affects – to 'grow' as Angela put it (Chapter 5) – reduce the bad. Modulating these affects, for capacitating bodies to act, should be at the heart of drug treatment and service provision. Second, following our relational ontology, our practices for knowing and intervening-with drugs have never been more important. Traditional boundaries between the service user and provider no longer hold. The 'other' is as much a part of 'us' as we are them. But this makes drug-service staffs' and systems' attentiveness and ability to respond to these treatment bodies paramount. Rather than privileging the autonomous (health choosing or even drug choosing) subject, this treatment practice and sensibility gets involved in these assemblages – in the tensions, attachments, flows and habits – to mediate or machine rather than free.

Treatment practices need to get closer to drug-using bodies and their relational forces to identify where power is made – where affects get materialised as thought, feeling and action. This could be explored through collaborative mapping tools. For example, when I asked participants how their lives and the services they received could be improved, their answers were rarely concerned with making changes to their drug use per se, but rather about obtaining *meaningful* employment and a safe and comfortable home. To map these desire flows and blockages holds more promise to find where specific empowerment and disempowerment occurs, and where to direct attention. Again, more than reducing harm, this is about improving bodies' capacities to act in their widest sense, whether this includes drugs or not.

Furthermore, treatment providers must increase their awareness over how they can 'block' bodies becoming-other, through regimes and regulations that structure people's days and wed them to the 'drug user' or worse still 'junkie' identity. I have provided several examples of such blockages throughout this book in relation to short opening times, strict opiate substitute regimes, disrespectful/stigmatising attitudes and an unwillingness to prescribe painkillers or opiate substitutes in emergency settings. These policies/technologies function to prevent people becoming employees, patients, students, sons, mothers, etc. We must, in drug services, make alternative 'becomings' possible, and open up 'lines of flight' through flexibile, creative and convenient care. Taking what Kane Race might call an 'affirmative approach to contingencies' (2018: 184), this is a call to be aware of how dis/empowerment is made in drug consumption and treatment events and thus to engender attentiveness and response-ability to bring about as many good affects and as few bad affects as possible irrespective of drug use. This is not a system of judging what is right or wrong from outside, but a speculative ethics of empowerment – to learn from and act on the relations we are to become.

As Sara Ahmed points out '"contingency" has the same root in Latin as the word "contact" (Latin: contingere: com-, with; tangere, to touch)' (2004: 28). Contingency then is linked to this onto-epistemological need to touch and be in touch. For drug treatment to be situated – a long established argument in the social sciences for/of harm reduction – it has to be contingent, that is to say, in touch. For example, Chapter 4 highlighted how experiences of addiction, far from being about an overpowering connection to a drug, were fundamentally linked to the legal system, institutions, knowledges and policies that meant participants lacked housing, a doctor, career, social network or prescription for their desired opiate substitute (which meant, for many, drug services had nothing to offer them). It is here that drug services fundamentally matter in how bodies come to matter, for in their rigid, one-size-fits-all approach they can limit, even harm bodies. Therefore, the kind of situated drug treatment advocated for here follows an ontological move to mattering which puts its own practices and attentiveness right at the centre of service users' health (capacity to affect and be affected). Such approach is able to respond to the many ways drugs can act, and treatment collectives (staff, technologies, policies, etc.) work *with* these enactments rather than acting to neglect or discipline them. For example, as we saw in the previous chapter, programmes that strive for opiate reductions fail to adapt to recipient's situated needs, making it too easy for them to fail, or rather, be failed. Technologies and services that lack response-ability risk becoming oppressive, 'fascist' spaces (Malins, 2017), where, as we have seen many participants, including perhaps even a worker, no longer wanted to be.[1]

Care and caring relationships in drug-service provision are often seen as something that occurs between the service user and provider – in care plans, key-working sessions, doctors' appointments, exchanging needles and syringes – but what this book has argued is that care is about much more than this. Feminists have long lamented the lack of attention that care has been given, especially the hidden care work – the behind the scenes, small acts of attention and maintenance for sustaining bodies and worlds. In reinvigorating Joan Tronto and Bernice Fischer's definition of care as '*everything that we do* to maintain, continue and repair "our world" (Tronto, 1993) so that we can live in it as well as possible', Puig de la Bellacasa (2017: 3) brings our attention to the many practices involved in holding relations together in our worldly becoming. She goes on: 'that world includes our bodies, ourselves, and our environment, *all of which we seek to interweave in a complex, life-sustaining web*' (2017: 3, original emphasis). This begs the question: What happens if we take all kinds of participants seriously – as participants in care?

In this study, care is shown in both people who inject drugs' and service providers' practices of working-with substances, licit and illicit, as well as other technologies, such as injecting equipment and assessment tools in an ethics of empowerment. This opens our thinking up to new kinds of care. I now wonder, for instance, what care (and exclusions) might be enacted in the 'recovery café' mentioned in Chapter 5, or in the increasing use of recovery groups I observed, like alternative therapies, exercise clubs, cooking and art workshops? But also, just as importantly and routinely overlooked, I now wonder what care is getting enacted in people's injecting practices? We saw how pleasure, for example, relied on a careful more-than-human balancing act of components and techno-corporeal techniques, but what happens if we also think of this embodiment as care-full? How are caring relations getting employed and felt in these enactments? How are these assemblages for pleasure also maintaining worlds? To widen out what is seen as care is to politicise where this care and attention is also not happening. What bodies are failed in our current attempts to care? What happens if we fail to respond to, or worse still, actively turn away from some bodies in their connections to drugs and drugged assemblages for becoming 'normal', 'healthy', sociable, relaxed, joyful, etc.? Rather than having predefined ideas of how to care and what is best for people as seen in some recovery-based programmes, we must actively and speculatively engage with bodies and problems as they emerge. Rather than a harm reduction 'from below' (Van Schipstal et al., 2016), this is a more-than-harm reduction *from within*.

Political reform

> It may be that a logic of care, and not a concern for reducing harms, offers the best hope for reform.
>
> Cameron Duff, 2015: 94

A policy focus on harm reduction is at risk of missing the many ways that drugs are engaged with for sustaining and enhancing life. Furthermore, as critiques of the 'war on drugs' mound, an alternate arbiter to harm is needed more than ever for global reform. For Cameron Duff, a 'logic of care', following an increasingly used human rights narrative (Jürgens et al., 2010) is best placed to serve this purpose (2015: 93). Here, I argue with Puig de la Bellacasa for a different logic of care that is fundamentally disentangled from the human subject or body. A care that originates from the sociomaterial collective as a speculative ethics of empowerment. I will first look at how this ethics challenges a moralist stance on prohibition, before looking at this alternative care as a 'minoritarian politics' and the 'people to come' (Deleuze and Guattari, 1987).

Policy advocates and politicians are increasingly willing to recognise that rather than reducing the harm of drug use, prohibition may actually be increasing the harms. And thus, paradoxically, if there is prohibition because drugs are dangerous, but drugs are made dangerous through prohibition, then who indeed is this war against? As philosopher of science, Isabelle Stengers, alerted us to many years ago:

> The categorization between legal and illegal has become the manifestation of the 'arbitrariness of the signifier', which is indifferent to reality since it is this that structures reality. And the law has finally become a project requiring not respect but adherence.
>
> (Stengers, 1997: 230)

Once 'the drug problem' has become a moral consensus in this way, it is no longer up for debate and controversy. This is what we have seen recently, for even though political lobbyists and politicians are more willing than ever to recognise prohibition as paradoxically harmful, little has changed. For example, commentators, eagerly awaiting the United Nations General Assembly Special Session (UNGASS) on 'the world drug problem' in 2016, convened by those governments most affected by the destructive effects of the illegal drug market, were bitterly disappointed to find global prohibition upheld (Fernandez Ochoa, 2016; Glenza, 2016). Here, I seek to contribute to a dismantling of this war on drugs; to stir up controversy and new ways of caring in and with policy.

'The logic of care', Duff says, 'would make care itself, and the promotion of health, the goals of drug policy rather than the prevention of use, or even the reduction of harm' (2015: 94). We are therefore arguing for the same thing, but the care revealed in becoming-with drug-using and injecting bodies in this book is a different kind of care. Rather than bringing care back to the self or individual, in which Duff, quoting Foucault (1997), says, 'the point is to establish a "certain relation to oneself"' (2015: 86), I want to broaden this out, as aforementioned, to a logic of care as collective. And, following Barad's notion of response-ability (noted above), I want to explore the ethico-political ramifications of these efforts as a 'minoritarian politics'.

A minoritarian politics, for Deleuze and Guattari (1987), is a politics concerned with attending to neglected things, people and relations, which gives rise to new ways of relating. 'Matters of care' are precisely about this minoritarian politics of attending to and assembling neglected things (Puig de la Bellacasa, 2017). Where Puig de la Bellacasa looks at soil as a multispecies world, as a system of maintenance rather than productivity, she is considering soil as a lively system that affects how humans relate to it and what they can become in being cared for back. This is an interdependency (rather than dependency as often conceived of in care work) that can be extended to injecting bodies and our capacity to care for them as always part of what they can become. A narrative of human rights or self-care risks turning care inwards towards the human or individual body ('bios'), where I hope to turn it outwards towards the collective work involved in living or becoming-minoritarian. This is a drug policy that asks: What changes can ensue if we take people's relationality seriously?

We saw how pleasure in Chapter 3 relied on an onto-epistemologically entangled 'success', in which citric acid, for example, was key to letting Lucy *know* that the injection had worked and could be enjoyed, without which she would be unsure and unmoved. A once facilitative substance for changing the chemical make-up of base heroin into a solution for injecting becomes an integral component of the embodied e/affect. To take this seriously is to be able to ask questions of public health policies that encourage vitamin c distribution over citric acid, as a milder acid for protecting vein health. This is not to suggest that these strategies are wrong, but to enable an approach that can better appreciate these bodily onto-epistemological concerns. That is to say, by being able to attend to these drug-body-world attachments, tensions, desires, and habits, we can redress a neglect of these relations integral but often seen as merely facilitative to bodies' becomings.

Policies must be open to the eventfulness of drugs and their effects. In this book, we have seen, for example: how drugged pleasures are contingent on assemblages of the substances, 'paraphernalia' and space-time; thoughts (about one's drug use) are entangled with the addiction concepts they plug into; and 'harms' or 'blockages' come about as toxic actants (like dirt) or stratifying bodies enter the injecting mix. It is only through more exacting interventions with these bodies that people who use drugs and drugs themselves can be imagined and done differently. Therefore, those policies most likely to succeed in potentialising better bodies (in their capacities to affect and be affected) are those that provide the necessary space for attachment-, tension-, desire- and habit-led treatment: to follow these relations between and beyond bodies, to see how boundaries are worked and reworked for better or worse, and to get involved in these processes.

Of course, this goes against a drug policy based on the drug as essentially bad, and furthermore, a care policy reliant on the human (given or not). As the former can now be agreed, I take up the latter. To reduce care to the human, even strategically, is to limit by design what care can be and do (Keane, 2003).[2] As previously stated, and highlighted throughout the chapters, care is a shared practice of empowerment performed by bodies, technologies and knowledges that involve us all. If we are ever to account for and respond to the multiple bodies brought into being in drug encounters, we must dislocate the individual, and this includes the self-caring one. By looking at care as a joint responsibility, a more tolerant approach of how drugs are part of living and keeping bodies together can evolve. In accepting that we live in complex bio-chemical-social worlds, we can *really* appreciate participants' concerns, for example, over recovery policies that mandate abstinence. This is not to say that these policies will not work for some people in some situations, but that our focus should always be on improving capacities to act more broadly (what Duff [2014a] calls 'assemblages of health'), whatever that may be. In this sense, care is a speculative ethics, as well as a non-normative and situational one, that cannot be decided in advance.

To be 'in touch', is also to be touched back (Barad, 2012; Puig de la Bellacasa, 2017). So, this call for heightened response-ability is also a plea to learn more from people who use drugs and their neglected attachments, tensions, flows and habits. This speaks to the reciprocity and interdependency (beyond dependency) at the heart of care and a politics of becoming-minoritarian – to be able to know and care for new bodies as the other within. It is in this sense that I advocate for an approach that gets closer to drugged bodies, to become drug users in this political sense. To get closer to these bodies is to be able to feel what it might be like to be affected by drugs in their assemblic make-up, so that to be open to the positive experiences is also to be able to know the many, and often overriding negative components, like those highlighted in Chapter 4, in being *known* as a drug user or worse 'junkie'.

By becoming-with injecting bodies, that is to say, minoritarian, in this way, we too (as readers, researchers, treatment providers, policymakers) are put at risk. Not only do injecting bodies destabilise our modes of knowing – our distinctions between nature/culture, subject/object, body/society, pleasure/addiction, normal/pathological – but our very being.

> Minorities, of course, are objectively definable states, states of language, ethnicity, or sex with their own ghetto territorialities, but they must also be thought of as seeds, crystals of becoming whose value is to trigger uncontrollable movements and deterritorializations of the mean or majority.
>
> (Deleuze and Guattari, 1987: 106)

Therefore, rather than advocating for people who use drugs to be moved closer to 'the human' as a 'majoritarian fact', with a given doctrine of rights, I call for a more radical political transformation.

> There is a majoritarian 'fact,' but it is the analytic fact of Nobody, as opposed to the becoming-minoritarian of everybody. That is why we must distinguish between: the majoritarian as a constant and homogeneous system [...] and the minoritarian as a potential, creative and created, becoming.
>
> (Deleuze and Guattari, 1987: 105–106)

Instead of pathologising and distancing people who use drugs from ourselves, to only then move them back towards us as 'humans' with a set of homogeneous rights, we need to do quite the opposite and get closer to them. It is towards this intimacy that policy should focus its attention. To be part of drug-using bodies in these fundamental ways, and for them to be part of us, is to embody this empathy in both directions, to care and be cared for.

Becoming drug users, or rather becoming-with drug-using bodies, we are better able to attune to their needs as the other within and learn from their experiences in potentialising new ways of living, not just with drugs, but more generally, which no longer depends on the binaries that these bodies disrupt: the autonomous, free, rational individual, 'in short, the average European [man], the subject of enunciation' (Deleuze and Guattari, 1987). As Colebrook notes: 'A minoritarian politics does not see itself as the expression of the people but as the creation of new peoples, a "people to come"' (2002: 63). This widening out of ourselves as collectives, as new peoples, in more-than-human worlds, offers a very different kind of ethico-political intervention than a biopolitics concerned with self-care.

I am interested in what new forms of becoming could emerge with policies concerned with care rather than harm. For example, Lancaster and colleagues (2017) show how a medicinal cannabis policy based on 'compassion' turned 'criminal' 'users' into 'patients' in need of 'care'. Something similar is occurring in the UK, in which the government has now legalised cannabis-derived medicinal products on prescription for some conditions (Home Office and Javid, 2018). This follows the high-profile cases of two (white) children with refractory epilepsy being denied such products known to alleviate their symptoms. But, again, this raises questions of how care is being rendered in these reforms and who is worthy of care and able to care (Farrugia et al, forthcoming; Gill et al., 2017; Martin et al., 2015). Although this likely reform feels far away from the kind of care that could benefit people who inject drugs, or lead to the de-criminalisation of all drugs, it may point towards drugs being judged more on their situational effects than their essentialised (and classed) chemical properties. I am therefore interested in how such policies can help to reconfigure our relationship to drugs and legitimise ways of living with drugs that are currently neglected, undermined, or worse still, punished.

Although non-normative, these drug policies of care, as I envisage, are by no means non-obligatory. Far from it, it is just that these obligations come from our collective learning and ability to respond from within rather than as a moral order from outside. Care, in this study, has emerged in various ways for doing bodies better: heroin (and crack cocaine) collectives worked to help participants walk, ease back pain, 'take the edge off', experience pleasure, 'do' the 'everyday'; and service provider collectives 'tinkered' with policies and tools in adapting to the specificity of bodies' situated needs. But in an ethico-political approach which also looks outwards, this is not just about the maintenance of more-than-human participant bodies, but a maintenance of networks beyond the body. Going against prohibition, a broader concept of care could extend to include the unregulated illegal markets and ecologies, which means opium eradication policies, brutal policing and environmental disasters (e.g. poppy blight) regularly disrupt the supply chain. For example, the heroin 'droughts' mentioned by participants are seen by the UK government to be a key reason for the rise in fatal opiate overdoses as the purity levels returned (PHE, 2017).

Following the previous sections on research and treatment, I call here for a heightened response-ability towards making policy and what policies can *do*. Reducing harm is only one, and, as conceived in public health, a particularly individualistic and anthropocentric way of doing care. So, whilst harm reduction is in many ways a matter of care, it is also a refrain on what care can be. I therefore advocate for a bigger imagining of care – which is less able to be brought back to the human body (as victim, perpetrator or protector):

> The point is not to dismiss the political importance of biosocialities but to argue for a displacement of ethopolitics in biopolitics that brings us closer to challenge what we include in bios as collective in search of as well as possible relationalities.
>
> (Puig de la Bellacasa, 2017: 140)

Dispersing agency and politics in this way offers more hope for increasing responsibility towards people who use drugs as we sensitise to the effects we have and our capacities to improve (and remove) relationalities.

In sum, then, by paying attention to injecting bodies rather than injecting (and drug-using) subjects and their objects, this book puts forward an approach to drug use that can more carefully and intimately pinpoint where and how, and to what effect, drug-body-worlds manifest and eventualise, and where to intervene. As care is always a mode of knowing and doing, it is perhaps misleading to separate out research, treatment and policy in this way. Nonetheless, I have found it useful to explore the many ways that we can be involved in this response-ablisation. Seeing these diverse research, treatment and policy practices as matters of care is crucial for reinvigorating an ethico-political approach to drug use where in recent years, in the UK, as well as elsewhere, record numbers of injecting and drug-using bodies have been failing to matter in the most dramatic and literal way. More than ever, *our mattering practices matter*. It is my assertion that by becoming-with injecting and drug-using bodies, we are entangled in their power to act or not. Thus, in our response-ability to them, I have shown in this book how bodies are not only brought into being, held together and experienced *with* drugs, but can be intervened-with as part of a speculative ethics to make them better.

Notes

1 This links to a trend seen nationally as less people are receiving treatment (NDTMS, 2016; 2017).
2 See Moore and Fraser (2006) for a discussion of the strategic use of the neoliberal subject in drug policy.

Participant list

(I have changed names and altered/removed some details to protect ano-
nymity. Descriptions of ethnicity follow participants' own wording)

Ajay – thirty-three years old, black British, from London. Ajay injects
heroin most days into his femoral vein rather than his arms to 'hide' his
using from external view. He is in receipt of a buprenorphine prescription.
Ajay let slip a few times that he also deals. He was recruited through and
received services at Dunswell.

Angela – recovery worker, previously called substance misuse practitioner, at the Dunswell service. Angela was a qualified counsellor and had
worked in the drugs field for eight years.

Anita – thirty-five years old, second-generation British Bangladeshi, from
London. Anita was told about the study via word-of-mouth and used a different service to the recruiting sites. Anita regularly injects 'speedballs' and
describes 'working on the street' as a sex worker to 'get money'. She recently
'slowed right down' and injects speedballs (two 'bags' [see Appendix II] of
each heroin and crack) a couple of times a week. She talks of 'substituting'
her drug use with drinking alcohol. Anita receives a methadone prescription which she describes as her 'saviour'.

Callum – interim manager at the Dunswell service. Callum had a background in finance and had only recently moved into the drugs field to help
with data and financial management.

Carlos – twenty-nine years old, originally from Spain, moved to England/
London in 2004. Carlos started snorting and then injecting cocaine aged
thirteen, and smoking heroin aged fifteen to 'come down' from the cocaine.
Carlos injects six 'speedballs' a day, made up of one bag of heroin and one
bag of cocaine (apart from in the morning, when he had two of each). He
receives 40 ml of methadone, to be taken daily under supervision at the
chemist.

Crystal – forty years old, describes her ethnicity as mixed race, from east
England. Crystal lives in shared housing, but often stays with her partner,
Mike (also interviewed). At nineteen years old, Crystal started injecting
speed daily, and then heroin and crack cocaine. Enrolled in a clinical trial,

she injects diamorphine twice a day under supervision. She also continues to inject 'speedballs' into her femoral vein once to twice a week (one to two bags of both heroin and crack per injection).

Dimitri – forty-one years old, British, with Turkish parents, from London. Dimitri injects three to seven bags of heroin a day. He smokes crack cocaine 'occasionally', although this has started to 'creep its way back in' (smoking a few times in the past week). Dimitri receives a Subutex [see Appendix II] prescription of 12mg a day, but frequently took less. He was recruited through/receives services at Eastford.

Dr Green – General Practitioner (GP), specialist in drug and alcohol use. Dr Green is the borough lead for substance misuse.

Ed – thirty-eight years old, white British, from London, lives in hostel accommodation. Ed started injecting 'speedballs' aged seventeen. He injects one to two times a day (one to two bags of heroin and crack in each injection). Ed recently received a Drug Rehabilitation Requirement, court-ordering him to comply with drug treatment. He takes 40ml methadone under daily supervision.

Eva – recovery social worker at Dunswell service. Eva has worked in the drugs field for five years.

Grigor – thirty-seven years old, Romanian. Grigor has been studying and working as an IT Engineer in London for the last thirteen years. I met with Grigor twice – at the Eastford service and then at the university. Grigor injects 'speedballs' multiple times a day (spending £100–200). He is court ordered, under a Drug Rehabilitation Requirement, to comply with drug treatment, including being prescribed 60ml methadone to be taken under daily supervision.

Gwen – forty-nine years old, white British, from London. Gwen looks after her grandchildren and works part-time as an artist. She owns her own flat. Gwen injects two bags of heroin a day, split two ways, between her and Sandra (also interviewed). She was recruited via word-of-mouth and was not attending any drug services as they could not prescribe her the opiate substitute, morphine, she wanted for her heroin use and chronic health conditions.

Jim – forty-five years old, white British, from London (with Scottish parents). Jim receives Employment Support Allowance (ESA) and lives in a hostel after having his council flat tenancy revoked. Enrolled in a clinical trial, he injects 200mg diamorphine and takes orally 40ml methadone twice a day under supervision. Up until recently, he was injecting three 'speedballs' a day (made up of three bags of heroin and three bags of crack cocaine), which has reduced to a few times a week. He drinks high-percentage beer every day.

Jon – thirty-seven years old, white British, from North England. Jon works part-time for a delivery company. He lives in his own flat. Jon started using opiates as a teenager when he worked for a chemist and stole pain medicine. He receives a 40ml methadone prescription and injects heroin every-so-often.

Karolina – When I first met Karolina, she had worked as a recover worker at the Eastford service for the last five years. She has since left the drugs field, and I interviewed her at the university.

Lucy – forty-two years old, white British, from south England. She volunteers for a charity and lives in her own council flat. Lucy started smoking and then injecting heroin in her early twenties. She finds it difficult to locate a vein, so injects only every-so-often (last injected a week ago), but smokes heroin (two bags) at least three times a week. She takes 50ml of prescribed methadone and 20mg of illicitly sought diazepam every day. Lucy was recruited through/received services at Eastford.

Malik – thirty-seven years old, describes his ethnicity as mixed race (Bangladeshi father, black British mother), from London. Malik started injecting speed at age nineteen, heroin in his early twenties, and crack in his early thirties. Malik smokes crack and injects heroin (one bag of each) once to twice a week. He is prescribed 50ml of methadone to be taken daily under supervision. He was recruited/receives services at Dunswell.

Mason – thirty-one years old, white British, from north England. Mason is street homeless. He injects two to three bags of heroin a day into his femoral vein. He is not attending any drug services. Mason was recruited through word-of-mouth and interviewed at the university.

Matias – fifty-six years old, South American. Matias injects one to three bags of heroin into his femoral vein every day. He receives Disability Living Allowance due to his poor mobility. Matias was recruited through word-of-mouth and attends a different drug service to Eastford/Dunswell. He is prescribed 35ml of methadone daily on a weekly take-home basis.

Matt – Assessor for residential rehabilitation and detox, based at the Dunswell service. Before this, Matt volunteered and worked for four years as a drug worker at the service.

Meg – forty-nine years old, white British/European (parents from Italy). She worked as a volunteer at a peer-led cooking group, and was in receipt of ESA. She lived in a hostel. Meg smoked crack cocaine daily and only injected heroin every-so-often. She has been prescribed methadone for the last twenty years, and received 45ml of methadone on a daily pickup basis. She was recruited through word-of-mouth and interviewed at the Eastford service.

Mike – thirty-four years old, white British, from London. Mike receives ESA and has a council tenancy. For the last nine months, he had been part of a diamorphine trial, and currently receives 150mg of diamorphine to be injected under supervision twice a day, and oral methadone. This had dramatically reduced his drug consumption. He injects 'speedballs' (one bag of heroin and crack) about once a week.

Mya – fifty-two years old, describes her ethnicity as mixed race, from London. Mya, like some others in the study recruited via word-of-mouth, was enrolled in a diamorphine trial. Prior to the trial, she had bought diamorphine privately through doctors and on the street. She injects 180ml of diamorphine and drinks 70ml of methadone under supervision in a clinic every day and is prescribed a further 50ml of methadone to take at home.

Nadiya – forty-four years old, Eastern European, moved to London twenty years ago. Nadiya works part-time as a cleaner. She first used heroin in her late twenties, stating that drugs weren't really her thing. Nadiya smokes heroin every two to three days, and injects occasionally. She is prescribed 40ml of methadone to be taken under daily supervision. She was recruited via word-of-mouth and attends a different service to Dunswell/Eastford.

Nyundo – Manager of the Eastford service. Nyundo previously worked for eight years as a Drug Intervention Programme (DIP) worker in the criminal justice system.

Paula – sixty years old, white British, from London. Paula's daughter lives with her and she helps to care for her grandchildren. Paula smokes crack (one bag approximately) once a week with friends, snorts cocaine at parties and 'speedballs' every-so-often. She was recruited through word-of-mouth. Her drug use had vastly reduced and she does not attend a drug service.

Phil – Council commissioner of drug and alcohol services. Phil had worked in the drugs field for many years following his own drug use issues.

Reggie – thirty-two years old, black British, from London. Reggie came into the Dunswell service with Ajay and saw the poster. Reggie started using crack and heroin aged thirteen. He smokes crack and injects 'speedballs' several times a day. Reggie is not receiving drug services or any substitute medication.

Sandra – forty-eight years old, white British, from north England. Sandra 'ran away' to London aged fifteen. Sandra buys and uses heroin with her friend, Gwen. She injects heroin in her femoral vein twice a day. Sandra lives in a hostel and receives ESA. She was on probation. She does not receive an opiate substitute.

Silvie – forty-four years old, white European, moved to England from Malta. Silvie works part-time as an office administrator. She started smoking heroin and crack in her early thirties. Silvie injects 'speedballs' (one bag of each heroin and crack) three to four times a day. She buys illicit methadone when she cannot source/afford heroin. Silvie was recruited via word-of-mouth and does not receive any drug services. I interviewed her at the university.

Simon – forty-four years old, white British, from south England, moved to London aged sixteen. Simon lives with his girlfriend. He smokes at least two bags of heroin a day, and injects when he can find a vein (once a month).

Simon receives 70ml of methadone daily. He drinks alcohol every day. He was recruited via word-of-mouth and attends a different service to Eastford/ Dunswell.

Simone – project leader at Dunswell. Simone has worked in the drugs field for ten years.

Suzy – forty-eight years old, white British, from London. Suzy had fifteen years of abstinence and worked in a rehabilitation centre. She relapsed a few years ago. Suzy injects three bags of heroin into her femoral vein and smokes crack cocaine. She picks up 40ml of methadone every day from the chemist, but only takes 25ml of it.

Sue – fifty-four years old, white British, from west England. Sue is a carer to her disabled son. From the early nineties, Sue injected heroin and 'speed-balls' every day, with periods of abstinence only when in prison. She is now trying not to use drugs, but 'slips up' every-so-often.

Tom – forty-seven years old, white British, from east England. I met Tom some months before the study started in a work setting. He kindly vol-unteered to 'pilot' the interview. Tom is employed part-time as a courier. He injects two to three bags (three to four injections) of heroin a day. Tom has been on and off opiate substitute treatment since his thirties, and is currently prescribed 45ml methadone a day, on a weekly take-home basis.

Vicki – fifty-four years old, white British, from the Midlands. Vicki works part-time in a restaurant. Since being enrolled on a diamorphine programme, she has stopped illicit heroin use and injects 140mg of diamor-phine every day under supervision and is prescribed 80ml of methadone.

Participant terminology

Bag (of heroin/crack) – heroin and crack cocaine are sold in small wraps, often referred to as bags. These contain roughly 0.1g each and are sold at £10. This is enough for one injection, although some people might use more than this and others might divide it across more than one injection. Dealers will frequently sell two bags for £15, or three bags for £20. It, therefore, often made sense for participants to 'pull' together to get these better offers.

Benzos – abbreviation of benzodiazepines, a group of tranquilliser pharmaceutical drugs, which includes diazepam (brand name, Valium).

Brown – heroin (its most common colour in the UK).

Buprenorphine (brand name, Subutex) – an opiate agonist, used in opiate substitution treatment (OST).

Clean – drug-free/abstinent. Although widely used, the term is considered derogatory and discouraged at services for perpetuating an image of drug users as dirty.

Clucking – withdrawing from heroin.

Cold turkey – to abstain from heroin with no support or opiate substitute. People may use diazepam to ease the pain.

Cook/ing up – turning 'base' heroin (how it is most commonly bought in the UK) into a soluble form for injecting by heating it up with water and a little acid (citric acid or vitamin c are supplied at needle exchanges).

Crack house – a flat where crack and heroin (predominantly) are bought and consumed.

Diamorphine – pharmaceutical-grade heroin, prescribed/acquired illicitly through a clinician.

Fix/ing – injection/injecting.

Gear – heroin.

Gouch – relaxing effects of heroin, which may lead to consumers dropping their head, slowing their speech and perhaps closing their eyes without being asleep.

Hit – injection, but also used to refer to the sudden high that an injection can produce.

Junkie – derogatory term for somebody who uses heroin.

Kicked it/the habit – abstaining from drug use, often heroin.

Methadone – a widely prescribed opiate (full opioid receptor agonist) used in opiate substitution treatment/therapy (OST). Most people in the UK can access OST (commonly methadone or buprenorphine) through their General Practitioner (GP) or at a drug service once they have evidenced (provided a positive drug test) for opiate use.

Needle exchange – a service that provides sterile needles, syringes and other injecting equipment such as alcohol swabs, citric acid, vitamin C, ampules of water and 'sharps bins'. It also disposes of returned needles and sharps bins.

Nicked – arrested by the police.

Old Bill – police.

Pins – needles/syringes.

Scoring – buying drugs.

Script –abbreviation of prescription, often referring to the opiate substitutes, methadone or buprenorphine.

Speedball – injecting heroin and crack cocaine together in the same injection. Crack cocaine is stirred into the solution once heroin has been turned into a soluble (by adding water, acid and heating). Sometimes also called 'snowballs'.

Subutex (see buprenorphine above).

Subuxone – a less frequently prescribed version of buprenorphine that has been manufactured with naloxone to prevent 'misuse'. The naloxone will cause withdrawal symptoms if injected.

Valium – brand name for diazepam, a tranquiller. Sometimes people refer to 'benzos' instead (above).

White – crack cocaine (its colour).

Appendix III

Body maps

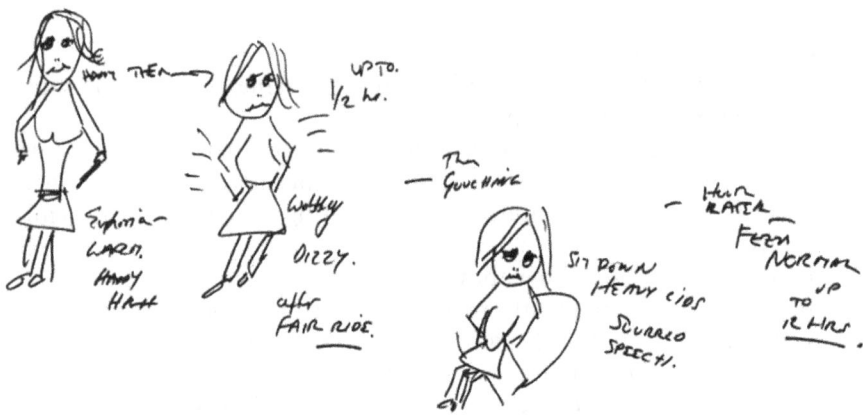

Figure A.1 Gwen's body map.

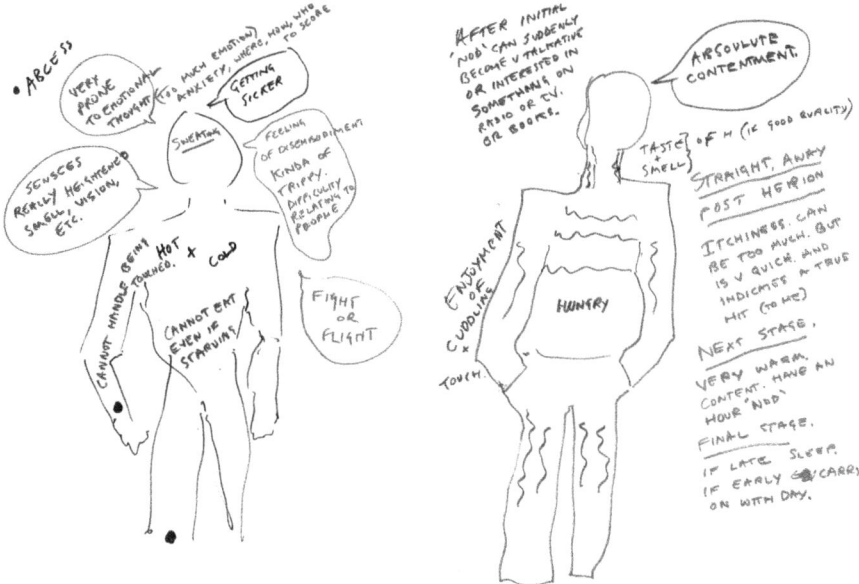

Figure A.2 Simon's body map.

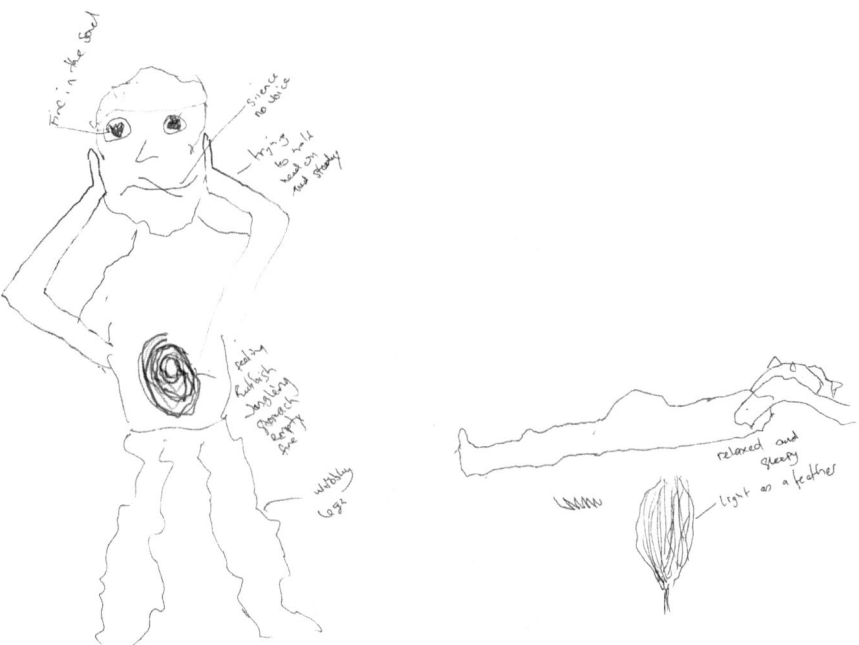

Figure A.3 Mason's body map.

Bibliography

ACDM (Advisory Council on the Misuse of Drugs). (2016) Reducing opioid-related deaths in the UK. Available at: https://www.gov.uk/government/publications/reducing-opioid-related-deaths-in-the-uk

Adkins, L. and Lury, C. (2009) Introduction: what is the empirical? *European Journal of Social Theory* 12(1): 5–20.

Ahmed, S. (2003) In the name of love. *Borderlands e-Journal*. Available at: www.borderlands.net.au/vol2no3_2003/ahmed_love.htm

Ahmed, S. (2004) *The cultural politics of emotion*. Edinburgh: Edinburgh University Press.

Aldridge, J., Measham, F. and Williams, L. (2011) *Illegal leisure revisited: changing patterns of alcohol and drug use in adolescents and young adults*. London: Routledge.

American Psychiatric Association. (2013) *Diagnostic and statistical manual of mental disorders* (5th ed.). Arlington, VA: American Psychiatric Publishing.

Anderson, B. and Tolia-Kelly, D. (2004) Matter(s) in social and cultural geography. *Geoforum* 35: 669–674.

Anderson, B. and Wylie, J. (2009) On geography and materiality. *Environment and Planning A* 41: 318–335.

Art2Be (no date) Art2Be [website]. Available at: http://art2bebodymaps.com/

Askew, R. (2016) Functional fun: legitimising adult recreational drug use. *International Journal of Drug Policy* 36: 112–119.

Bacchi, C. (2009) *Analysing policy: what's the problem represented to be?* Frenchs Forest, NSW: Pearson Australia.

Bacchi, C. (2012) Why study problematizations? Making politics visible. *Open Journal of Political Science* 2(1): 1–8.

Back, L. (2012) Live sociology: social research and its futures. In L. Back and N. Puwar (Eds) *Live methods*. Malden, MA: Wiley-Blackwell. Pp 18–39.

Back, L. and Puwar, N. (2012) *Live methods*. Malden, MA: Wiley-Blackwell.

Barad, K. (2003) Posthumanist performativity: toward an understanding of how matter comes to matter. *Signs: Journal of Women in Culture & Society* 28(3): 801–830.

Barad, K. (2007) *Meeting the universe halfway: quantum physics and the entanglement of matter and meaning*. Durham; London: Duke University Press.

Barad, K. (2012) On Touching - the inhuman that therefore I am. *Differences: A Journal of Feminist Cultural Studies* 23(3): 206–223.

BBC (Producer) (2012, Aug 16) *Russell Brand: from addiction to recovery* [Television broadcast]. Available at: www.bbc.co.uk/programmes/p00wq21g

BBC (Producer) (2014, Dec15) *Russell Brand: end the drugs war* [Television broadcast]. Available at: www.bbc.co.uk/programmes/b04v2zrg

BBC Radio 4 (Producer) (2016, Aug 28) *Choose Life* [Audio podcast]. Available at: www.bbc.co.uk/programmes/b070hsc

Becker, H.S. (1953) Becoming a marihuana user. *American Journal of Sociology* 59(3): 235–242.

Bennett, J. (2010) *Vibrant matter: a political ecology of things.* Durham: Duke University Press.

Bennett, T. Dodsworth, F., Noble, G., Poovey, M. and Watkins, M. (2013) Habit and habituation: governance and the social. *Body & Society* 19(2–3): 3–29.

Bergschmidt, V.B. (2004) Pleasure, power and dangerous substances: applying Foucault to the study of 'heroin dependence' in Germany. *Anthropology and Medicine* 11(1): 59–73.

Berridge, K.C. and Robinson, T.E. (2016) Liking, wanting, and the incentive-sensitization theory of addiction. *American Psychology* 71(8): 670–679.

Berridge, K.C., Robinson, T.E. and Aldridge, J.W. (2010) Dissecting components of reward: 'liking', 'wanting', and learning. *Current Opinion in Pharmacology* 9(1): 65–73.

Berridge, V. (1999) Histories of harm reduction: illicit drugs, tobacco, and nicotine. *Substance Use and Misuse* 34(1): 35–47.

Berridge, V. (2012) The rise, fall, and revival of recovery in drug policy. *Lancet* 379: 22–33.

Biehl, J. (2010) Human pharmakon: symptoms, technologies, subjectivities. In B.J. Good, M.J. Fischer, S.S. Willen and M. DelVecchio (Eds) *A reader in medical anthropology.* Chichester: Wiley-Blackwell. Pp. 213–232.

Bjerg, O. (2008) Drug addiction and capitalism: too close to the body. *Body & Society* 14(2): 1–22.

Blackman, L. (2008) *The body: the key concepts.* Oxford; New York: Berg

Blackman, L. (2012) *Immaterial bodies: affect, embodiment, mediation.* London: Sage.

Blackman, L. (2013) Habit and affect: revitalizing a forgotten history. *Body & Society* 19(2–3): 186–216.

Blackman, L. and Venn, C. (2010) Affect. *Body & Society* 16(1): 7–28.

Bobel, C. (2010) *New Blood: third-wave feminism and the politics of menstruation.* New Brunswick; New Jersey; London: Rutgers University Press.

Bøhling, F. (2014) Crowded contexts: on the affective dynamics of alcohol and other drug use in nightlife spaces. *Contemporary Drug Problems* 41: 361–392.

Bøhling, F. (2017) Psychedelic pleasures: an affective understanding of the joys of tripping. *International Journal of Drug Policy* 49:133–143

Boothroyd, D. (2004) *Culture on drugs: narco-cultural studies of high modernity.* Manchester: Manchester University Press.

Bourgois, P. (1995) *In search of respect: selling crack in El Barrio.* Cambridge: Cambridge University Press.

Bourgois, P. (1998) The moral economies of homeless heroin addicts: confronting ethnography, HIV risk, and everyday violence in San Francisco shooting encampments. *Substance Use and Misuse* 33: 2323–2351.

Bourgois, P. (2000) Disciplining addictions: the bio-politics of methadone and heroin in the United States. *Culture, Medicine and Psychiatry* 24(2): 165–195.

Bourgois, P. and Schonberg, J. (2009) *Righteous dopefiend.* Berkeley; London: University of California Press.

Bowers, A.L. (2009) *'As un-American as rabies': addiction and identity in American postwar junkie literature* (Unpublished PhD thesis). Texas A&M University.

Boyt, A. (2014, Nov) Staying alive. *Drug and Drink News.* p. 7. Available at: www.drinkanddrugsnews.com

Brain, K. (2000) Youth, alcohol, and the emergence of the post-modern alcohol order. Institute of Alcohol Studies. Available at: www.isa.org.uk/iaspapers/bran paper.pdf

Bravo, M.J., Barrio, G., De La Fuente, L., Royuela, L., Domingo, L. and Silva, T. (2003) Reasons for selecting an initial route of heroin administration and for subsequent transitions during a severe HIV epidemic. *Addiction* 98(6): 749–760.

Brett-MacLean, P. (2009) Body mapping: embodying the self living with HIV/AIDS. *Canadian Medical Association Journal* 19(7): 140–141.

Bundy, H. and Quintero, G. (2017) From mundane medicines to euphorigenic drugs: how pharmaceutical pleasures are initiated, foregrounded, and made durable. *International Journal of Drug Policy* 49: 109–116.

Bunton, R. and Coveney, J. (2011) Drugs' pleasures. *Critical Public Health* 2(1): 19–23.

Buscher, M., Urry, J. and Witchger, K. (Eds) (2011) *Mobile methods.* Abington, Oxon: Routledge.

Carr, E.S. (2011) *Scripting addiction: the politics of therapeutic talk and American society.* Princeton; Oxford: Princeton University Press.

Channel 4 (2012) Drugs live: ecstasy trial. Available at: www.channel4.com/programmes/drugs-live/episode-guide/series-1

Clough, P.T. (2009) The new empiricism: affect and sociological method. *European Journal of Social Theory* 2: 43–61.

Clough, P.T. and Halley, J.O.M. (2007) *The affective turn: theorizing the social.* Durham: Duke University Press.

Colebrook, C. (2002) *Understanding Deleuze.* Crows Nest, NSW: Allen & Unwin.

Coleman, R. and Ringrose, J. (2013) *Deleuze and research methodologies.* Edinburgh: Edinburgh University Press.

Collin, M. (1996, Nov 13) Medicated followers of fashion. *Time Out.* p. 13.

Cooper, M. (2012) The pharmacology of distributed experiment – user-generated drug innovation. *Body & Society* 18(3–4): 18–43.

Coveney, J. and Bunton, R. (2003) In pursuit of the study of pleasure: implications for health research and practice. *Health* 7(2): 161–179.

CSJ (The Centre for Social Justice) (2013) *No quick fix: exposing the depth of Britain's drug and alcohol problem* [Online report]. Available at: www.centrefor socialjustice.org.uk/UserStorage/pdf/Pdf%20reports/addict.pdf

CSJ (The Centre for Social Justice) (2014) *Ambitious for recovery tackling drug and alcohol addiction in the UK* [Online report]. Available at: Www.Centreforsocial justice.Org.Uk/Userstorage/Pdf/Pdf%20reports/CSJJ2073_Addiction_15.08. 14_2.Pdf

Del Busso, L.A. and Reavey, P. (2013) Moving beyond the surface: a poststructuralist phenomenology of young women's embodied experiences in everyday life. *Psychology & Sexuality* 4(1): 46–61.

Deleuze, G. (1977) Desire and Pleasure. In D. Lapoujade (Ed) (2006) *Two regimes of madness: texts and interviews 1975–1995.* New York; Los Angeles, CA: Semiotext(e). Pp. 122–135.

Deleuze, G. (1978) Two questions on drugs. In D. Lapoujade (Ed) (2006) *Two regimes of madness: Texts and interviews 1975–1995.* Los Angeles, CA; New York: Semiotext(e). Pp. 151–156.

Deleuze, G. (1990) *The logic of sense.* New York: Columbia University Press.

Deleuze, G. (1992) *Expressionism in philosophy: Spinoza.* New York: Zone Books.

Deleuze, G. (1994) *Difference and repetition.* New York: Columbia University Press.

Deleuze, G. (1995a) Immanence: a life. In D. Lapoujade (Ed) (2006) Two regimes of madness: Texts and interviews 1975–1995. Los Angeles, CA; New York: Semiotext(e). Pp. 384–391.

Deleuze, G. (1995b) *Negotiations.* New York: Columbia University Press.

Deleuze, G. (2001) *Pure immanence: essays on a life.* New York: Zone books.

Deleuze, G. (2006) Desire and pleasure. In *Two regimes of madness: texts and interviews 1975–1995.* New York: Semiotext(e). Pp. 122–134.

Deleuze, G. and Guattari, F. (1983) *Anti-oedipus: capitalism and schizophrenia.* Minneapolis: University of Minnesota Press.

Deleuze, G. and Guattari, F. (1987) *A thousand plateaus: capitalism and schizophrenia.* Minneapolis; London: University of Minnesota Press.

Deleuze, G. and Guattari, F. (1994) *What is philosophy?* New York: Columbia University Press.

Deleuze, G. and Parnet, C. (2007) *Dialogues II. Revised edition.* New York: Columbia University Press.

Demant, J. (2009) When alcohol acts: an actor-network approach to teenagers, alcohol and parties. *Body & Society* 15(1): 25–46.

Demant, J. (2013) Affected in the nightclub: a case study of regular clubbers' conflictual practices in nightclubs. *International Journal of Drug Policy* 24(3): 196–202.

Demant, J., Ravn, S. and Thorsen, K. (2010) Club studies: methodological perspectives for researching drug use in a central youth social space. *Leisure Studies* 29(3): 241–252.

Dennis, F. (2016) Encountering 'triggers': drug-body-world entanglements of injecting drug use. *Contemporary Drug Problems* 43(2): 126–141.

Dennis, F. (forthcoming) Body-mapping as 'allegory': 'relating to' drug-using bodies. *Body & Society.*

Dennis, F. and Farrugia, A. (2017) Materialising drugged pleasures: practice, politics, care. *International Journal of drug Policy* 49: 86–91.

Despret, V. (2004) The body we care for: figures of anthropo-zoo-genesis. *Body & Society* 10(2–3): 111–134.

Despret, V. (2013) Responding bodies and partial affinities in human–animal worlds. *Theory, Culture & Society* 30(7–8): 51–76.

Dilkes-Frayne, E. (2014) Tracing the 'event' of drug use: 'context' and the coproduction of a night out on MDMA. *Contemporary Drug Problems* 41(3): 445–479.

Dilkes-Frayne, E. and Duff, C. (2017) Tendencies and trajectories: the production of subjectivity in an event of drug consumption. *Environment and Planning D: Society and Space* 35(5): 951–967.

Dilkes-Frayne, E., Fraser, S., Pienaar, K. and Kokanovic, R. (2017) Iterating 'addiction': residential relocation and the spatio-temporal production of alcohol and other drug consumption patterns. *International Journal of Drug Policy* 44: 164–173.

Dodsworth, F.M. (2013) Habit, the criminal body and the body politic in England, c.1700–1800. *Body & Society* 19(2–3): 83–106.

Domínguez Rubio, F. (2016) On the discrepancy between objects and things: an ecological approach. *Journal of Material Culture* 21(1) 59–86.

Dorrell, J. (2007) Using 'body mapping' to flag workers' ill health. Available at: www.healthandsafetyatwork.com/hsw/content/using-body-mapping-flag-workers-ill-health

Drumm, R.D., McBride, D., Metsch, L., Neufeld, M. and Sawatsky, A. (2005) 'I'm a health nut!" street drug users' accounts of self-care strategies. *Journal of Drug Issues* 35: 607–629.

Duff, C. (2007) Towards a theory of drug use contexts: space, embodiment and practice. *Addiction Research & Theory* 15(5): 503–519.

Duff, C. (2009) The drifting city: the role of affect and repair in the development of 'enabling environments'. *International Journal of Drug Policy* 20(3): 202–208.

Duff, C. (2011) Reassembling (social) contexts: new directions for a sociology of drugs. *International Journal of Drug Policy* 22(6): 404–406.

Duff, C. (2012) Accounting for context: exploring the role of objects and spaces in the consumption of alcohol and other drugs. *Social & Cultural Geography* 13(2): 145–159.

Duff, C. (2013) The social life of drugs. *International Journal of Drug Policy* 24(3): 167–172.

Duff, C. (2014a) *Assemblages of health: Deleuze's empiricism and the ethology of life.* London; New York: Springer.

Duff, C. (2014b) The place and time of drugs. *International Journal of Drug Policy* 25(3): 633–639.

Duff, C. (2015) Governing drug use otherwise: for an ethics of care. *Journal of Sociology* 51(1): 81–96.

Duff, C. (2017) Critical drug studies after the ontological turn [unpublished conference paper]. *Contemporary Drug Problems Conference 2017.* Pp. 23–25 Aug, Helsinki.

Duff, C. (2018) A new empiricism for harm reduction. *International Journal of Drug Policy* 61: 59–61.

Duff, C. and Moore, D. (2015) Going out, getting about: atmospheres of mobility in Melbourne's night-time economy. *Social & Cultural Geography* 16(3): 299–314.

Duke, K., Herring, R., Thickett, A., Thom, B. (2013) Substitution treatment in the era of 'recovery': an analysis of stakeholder roles and policy windows in Britain. *Substance Use & Misuse* 48: 966–976.

Dumit, J. (2012) *Drugs for life: how pharmaceutical companies define our health.* Durham: Duke University Press.

Duncan, T., Duff, C., Sebar, B. and Lee, J. (2017) 'Enjoying the kick': locating pleasure within the drug consumption room. *International Journal of Drug Policy* 49: 92–101.

Dwyer, R. (2008) Privileging pleasure: temazepam injection in a heroin market place. *International Journal of Drug Policy* 19(5): 367–374.

Dwyer, R. and Moore, D. (2013) Enacting multiple methamphetamines: the ontological politics of public discourse and consumer accounts of a drug and its effects. *International Journal of Drug Policy* 24(3): 203–211.

Eagles, J. (2015) *Blood illuminations* [Art installation]. Available at: http://jordan eagles.com

Erickson, P., Riley, D., Cheung, Y. and O'Hare, P. (1997) *Harm reduction: a new direction for drug policies and programs.* Toronto, ON: University of Toronto Press.

Farrugia, A. (2015) 'You can't just give your best mate a massive hug every day': young men, play and MDMA. *Contemporary Drug Problems* 42(3): 240–256.

Farrugia, A., Fraser, S., Dwyer, R., Renae, F., Neale, J., Dietze, P., and Strang, J. S. (2019) Take-home naloxone and the politics of care. *Sociology of Health and Illness.* (Accepted/In press).

Featherstone, M. (1991) The body in consumer culture. In B. Turner (Ed) *The body: social process and cultural theory.* London: Sage Publications. Pp. 170–197.

Fernandez Ochoa, J. (2016, 3 May) After UNGASS 2016: Disappointment and resolve (blog post). Available at: https://idpc.net/blog/2016/05/UNGASS2016-disappointement-and-resolve

Fischer, B., Turnbull, S., Poland, B. and Haydon, E. (2004) Drug use, risk and urban order: examining supervised injection sites (SISs) as 'governmentality'. *International Journal of Drug Policy* 15: 357–365.

Fitzgerald, J.L. (1998) An assemblage of desire, drugs and techno. *Angelaki: Journal of the Theoretical Humanities* 3(2): 41.

Fitzgerald, J.L. (2015) *Framing drug use: bodies, space, economy and crime.* Basingstoke: Palgrave Macmillan.

Fitzgerald, J.L. and Threadgold, T. (2004) Fear of sense in the street heroin market. *International Journal of Drug Policy* 15(5–6): 407–417.

Fitzgerald, J.L. and Threadgold, T. (2007) Desire and the abject in the city becoming-other. *Cultural Studies Review* 13(1) 105–120.

Foucault, M. (1977) *Discipline and punish: the birth of the prison.* London: Penguin.

Foucault, M. (1997) On the genealogy of ethics: an overview of work in progress. In P. Rabinow (Ed) *The essential works of Michel Foucault*, vol. 1. London: New Press. Pp. 253–80.

Fraser, M. (2010) Facts, ethics and event. In C. Bruun Jensen and K. Ro"dje (Eds) *Deleuzian intersections in science, technology and anthropology.* New York: Berghahn Press. Pp. 57–82.

Fraser, S. (2004) 'It's your life!': Injecting drug users, individual responsibility and hepatitis C prevention. *Health: An Interdisciplinary Journal for the Social Study of Health, Illness and Medicine* 8(2): 199–221.

Fraser, S. (2006) The chronotope of the queue: methadone maintenance treatment and the production of time, space and subjects. *International Journal of Drug Policy* 17(3): 192–202.

Fraser, S. (2013) The missing mass of morality: a new fitpack design for hepatitis C prevention in sexual partnerships. *International Journal of Drug Policy* 24(3): 212–219.

Fraser, S. (2016) Articulating addiction in alcohol and other drug policy: a multiverse of habits. *International Journal of Drug Policy* 31: 6–14.

Fraser, S., Hopwood, M., Treloar, C. and Brener, L. (2004) Needle fictions: medical constructions of needle fixation and the injecting drug user. *Addiction Research & Theory* 12(1): 67–76.

Fraser, S., Moore, D. and Keane, H. (2014) *Habits: remaking addiction.* Basingstoke: Palgrave Macmillan.

Fraser, S. and Moore, D. (Eds) (2011) *The drug effect: health, crime and society.* Cambridge: Cambridge University Press.

Fraser, S. and Treloar, C. (2006) 'Spoiled identity' in hepatitis C infection: the binary logic of despair. *Critical Public Health* 16(2): 99–110.

Fraser, S., Treloar, C., Gendera, S. and Rance, J. (2017) 'Affording' new approaches to couples who inject drugs: a novel fitpack design for hepatitis C prevention. *International Journal of Drug Policy* 50: 19–35.

Fraser, S. and valentine, k. (2006) 'Making blood flow': materializing blood in body modification and blood-borne virus prevention. *Body & Society* 12(1): 97–119.

Fraser, S. and valentine, k. (2008) *Substance and substitution: methadone subjects in liberal societies.* Basingstoke: Palgrave Macmillan.

Fraser, S., valentine, k. and Roberts, C. (2009) Living drugs. *Science as Culture* 18(2): 123–131.

Friedman, J. and Alicea, M. (2001) *Surviving heroin: interviews with women in methadone clinics.* Gainesville: University Press of Florida.

Fry, M. (2011) Seeking the pleasure zone: understanding young adult's intoxication culture. Australasian. *Marketing Journal* 19: 65–70.

Fusco, C. (2008) 'Naked truths'? Ethnographic dilemmas of doing research on the body in social spaces. In K. Gallagher (Ed) *The methodological dilemma: creative, critical and collaborative approaches to qualitative research.* Abingdon, Oxon; New York: Routledge. Pp. 159–185.

Gastaldo, D., Magalhães, L., Carrasco, C. and Davy, C. (2012) Body-map storytelling as research: methodological considerations for telling the stories of undocumented workers through body mapping. Available at: www.migrationhealth.ca/undocumented-workers-ontario/body-mapping

Gauntlett, D. (2007) *Creative explorations: new approaches to identities and audiences.* London: Routledge.

Giddings, D., Christo, G. and Davy, J. (2003) Reasons for injecting and not injecting: a qualitative study to inform therapeutic intervention. *Drugs: Education, Prevention and Policy* 10(1): 95–104.

Gill, N., Singleton, V. and Waterton, C. (Eds) (2017) *Care and policy practices.* Dorchester: Sociological Review Monographs.

Gilroy, P. (2005) Could you be loved? Bob Marley, anti-politics and universal sufferation. *Critical Quarterly* 47(1): 226–245.

Glenza, J. (2016, Apr 20) UN backs prohibitionist drug policies despite call for more 'humane solution'. *The Guardian.* Available at: www.theguardian.com/world/2016/apr/19/un-summit-global-war-drugs-agreement-approved

Gomart, E. (2002a) Towards generous constraint: freedom and coercion in a French addiction treatment. *Sociology of Health & Illness* 24(5): 517–549.

Gomart, E. (2002b) Methadone: six effects in search of a substance. *Social Studies of Science* 32(1): 93–135.

Gomart, E. (2004) Surprised by methadone: in praise of drug substitution treatment in a French clinic. *Body & Society* 10(2–3): 85–110.

Gomart, E. and Hennion, A. (1999) A sociology of attachment: music amateurs, drug users. In J. Law and J. Hassard (Eds) *Actor network theory and after.* Oxford: Blackwell/Sociological Review. Pp. 220–248.

Gonçalves, D.M., Kolstee, J., Ryan, D. and Race, K. (2016) Harm reduction in process: the ACON Rovers, GHB, and the art of paying attention. *Contemporary Drug Problems* 43(4) 314–330.

Gowan, T., Whetstone, S. and Andic, T. (2012) Addiction, agency, and the politics of self-control: doing harm reduction in a heroin users' group. *Social Science & Medicine* 74(8): 1251–1260.

Green, R. and Moore, D. (2009) 'Kiddie drugs' and controlled pleasure: recreational use of dexamphetamine in a social network of young Australians. *International Journal of Drug Policy* 20(5): 402–408.

Grosz, E. (2013) Habit today: Ravaisson, Bergson, Deleuze and us. *Body & Society* 19(2–3): 217–239.

Guillaume, L. and Hughes, J. (Eds) (2011) *Deleuze and the body.* Edinburgh: Edinburgh University Press.

Hamilton, I. and Stevens, A. (2017, Nov 9) Drug deaths increase as fewer people access treatment. Available at: https://theconversation.com/drug-deaths-increase-as-fewer-people-access-treatment-84784

Hamilton, I. and Stevens, A. (2018, Aug 6) Record level of drug deaths in England and Wales – latest official figures. Available at: https://theconversation.com/record-level-of-drug-deaths-in-england-and-wales-latest-official-figures-99710

Haraway, D.J. (1991a) Situated knowledges: the science question in feminism and the priviledge of partial perspective. In D.J. Haraway (Eds) *Simians, cyborgs, and women: the reinvention of nature.* London: Free Association Books. Pp. 183–203.

Haraway, D.J. (1991b) The biopolitics of postmodern bodies: constitutions of self in immune system discourse. In D.J. Haraway (Eds) *Simians, cyborgs and women: the reinvention of nature.* London: Free Association Books. Pp. 203–231.

Haraway, D.J. (1997) *Modest_Witness@Second_Millenium: FemaleMan_Meets_OncoMouse: Feminism and Technoscience.* New York: Routledge.

Haraway, D.J. (2003) *The companion species manifesto: dogs, people, and significant otherness.* Chicago, IL: Prickly Paradigm Press.

Haraway, D.J. (2008) *When species meet.* Minneapolis: University of Minnesota Press.

Haraway, D.J. (2013) Sowing worlds: a seed bag for terraforming with earth others. In M. Grebowicz and H. Merrick (Eds) *Beyond the cyborg: adventures with Donna Haraway.* New York: Columbia University Press. Pp. 137–147.

Haraway, D.J. (2016) *Staying with the trouble: making kin in the chthulucene.* Durham: Duke University Press.

Harris, M. (2005) Living with hepatitis C: the medical encounter. *New Zealand Sociology* 20(1): 4–19.

Harris, M. (2009) Injecting, infection, illness: abjection and hepatitis C stigma. *Body & Society* 15(4): 33–51.

Harris, M. (2015) 'Three in the room': embodiment, disclosure, and vulnerability in qualitative research. *Qualitative Health Research* 25(12): 1689–1699.

Harris, M. and Rhodes, T. (2012) Venous access and care: harnessing pragmatics in harm reduction for people who inject drugs. *Addiction* 107(6): 1090–1096.

Harris, M. and Rhodes, T. (2013a) Methadone diversion as a protective strategy: the harm reduction potential of 'generous constraints'. *International Journal of Drug Policy* 24(6): 43–50.

Harris, M. and Rhodes, T. (2013b) Hepatitis C treatment access and uptake for people who inject drugs: a review mapping the role of social factors. *Harm Reduction Journal* 10: 7–20.

Hart, A. (2018) Making a difference? Applying Vitellone's Social Science of the Syringe to performance and image enhancing drug injecting. *International Journal of Drug Policy* 61: 69–73.

Heather, N., Wodak, A., Nadelmann, E. and O'Hare, P. (Eds) (1993) *Psychoactive drugs and harm reduction: from faith to science*. London: Whurr.

Henare, A.J.M., Holbraad, M. and Wastell, S. (Eds) (2007) *Thinking through things: theorising artefacts ethnographically*. London; New York: Routledge

Hennion, A. (2001) Music lovers. Taste as performance. *Theory, Culture & Society* 18 (5): 1–22.

Hennion A (2003) Music and mediation: towards a new sociology of music. In M. Clayton, T. Herbert and R. Middleton (Eds) *The Cultural Study of Music*. London: Routledge. Pp 80–91.

Hennion, A. (2007) Those things that hold us together: taste and sociology. *Cultural Sociology* 1(1): 97–114.

Hennion, A. (2012, Sept 9–21) Attachments: a pragmatist view of what holds us [Online conference paper]. *The first European pragmatism conference Roma*. Available at: www.nordprag.org/papers/epc1/Hennion.pdf

Hennion, A., Maisonneuve, S. and Gomart, E. (2000) *Figures de l'amateur: formes, objets et pratiques de l'amour de la musique d'aujourd'hui*. Paris: La Documentation Française.

Hickey-Moody, A. (2013) Affect as method: feelings, aesthetics and affective pedagogy. In R. Coleman and J. Ringrose (Eds) *Deleuze and research methodologies*. Edinburgh: Edinburgh University Press. Pp. 79–96.

HM Government (2015) Drug strategy 2010: a balanced approach. Third annual review. Available at: www.gov.uk/government/uploads/system/uploads/attachment_data/file/407334/Cross-Government_Drug_Strategy_Annual_Review.pdf

Home Office (2010) *Drug strategy 2010: Reducing demand, restricting supply, building recovery: supporting people to live a drug free life*. London: Home Office.

Home Office (2012) *Putting full recovery first*. London: Home Office.

Home Office (2017) *2017 Drug strategy*. London: Home Office.

Home Office and Javid, S. (2018) Government announces that medicinal cannabis is legal. Available at: www.gov.uk/government/news/government-announces-that-medicinal-cannabis-is-legal

Hussey, A. (2014) *The long tradition of drug use in creativity*. BBC Radio 4. Available at: www.bbc.co.uk/programmes/p01q06cm

Hutton, F. (2012) Harm reduction, students and pleasure: an examination of student responses to a binge drinking campaign. *International Journal of Drug Policy* 23(3): 229–235.

IHRA (International Harm Reduction Association) (2010) *What is Harm Reduction? A position statement from the International Harm Reduction Association*. Available at: www.ihra.net/what-is-harm-reduction.

INPUD (The International Network of People Who Use Drugs) (2015) *Response to Russell Brand's documentary, 'Russell Brand: End the War on Drugs'.* Available at: www.inpud.net/en/news/open-letter-russell-brand-end-war-drugs

Ivsins, A. and Marsh, S. (2018) Exploring what shapes injection and non-injection among a sample of marginalized people who use drugs. *International Journal of Drug Policy* 57: 72–78.

Jackson, A.Y and Mazzei, L.A. (2012) *Thinking with theory in qualitative research: viewing data across multiple perspectives.* London; New York: Routledge.

Jackson, P. (2000) Rematerializing social and cultural geography. *Social and Cultural Geography* 1: 9–14.

Jürgens, R.J., Csete, J.J., Amon, S., Baral, C. and Beyrer, C. (2010) People who use drugs, HIV, and human rights. *The Lancet* 376(9739): 475–485.

Keane, H. (2002) *What's wrong with addiction?* New York: New York University Press.

Keane, H. (2003) Critiques of harm reduction, morality and the promise of human rights. *International Journal of Drug Policy* 14: 227–232.

Keane, H. (2009) Foucault on methadone: beyond biopower. *International Journal of Drug Policy* 20: 450–452.

Krarup, T.M. and Blok, A. (2011) Unfolding the social: quasi-actants, virtual theory, and the new empiricism of Bruno Latour. *The Sociological Review* 59(1): 42–63.

Kristeva, J. (1982) *Powers of horror: an essay on abjection.* New York: Columbia University Press.

Lancaster, K., Duke, K. and Ritter, A. (2015) Producing the 'problem of drugs': a cross national-comparison of 'recovery' discourse in two Australian and British reports. *International Journal of Drug Policy* 26(7): 617–625.

Lancaster, K., Seear, K. and Ritter, A. (2017) Making medicine; producing pleasure: a critical examination of medicinal cannabis policy and law in Victoria, Australia. *International Journal of Drug Policy* 49: 117–125.

Latimer, J. (2013) Being alongside: rethinking relations amongst different kinds. *Theory, Culture & Society* 30: 77–104.

Latimer, J. and Miele, M. (2013) Naturecultures? Science, affect and the non-human. *Theory, Culture & Society* 30(7–8): 5–31.

Latour, B. (1987) *Science in action.* Cambridge, MA: Harvard University Press.

Latour, B. (1988) *The pasteurization of France.* Cambridge, MA: Harvard University Press.

Latour, B. (1993) *We have never been modern.* Cambridge, MA: Harvard University Press.

Latour, B. (1999a) Factures/fractures: from the concept of network to the concept of attachment. *RES: Anthropology and Aesthetics* 36: 20–31.

Latour, B. (1999b) Pandora's hope: essays on the reality of science studies. Cambridge, MA; London: Harvard University Press.

Latour, B. (2000) When things strike back: a possible contribution of 'science studies' to the social sciences. *The British Journal of Sociology* 51(1): 107–123.

Latour, B. (2004a) How to talk about the body? The normative dimension of science studies. *Body & Society* 10: 205–229.

Latour (2004b) *Politics of nature: how to bring the sciences into democracy.* Cambridge, MA: Harvard University Press.

Latour, B. (2005a) *Reassembling the social: an introduction to actor-network-theory.* Oxford: Oxford University Press.

Latour, B. (2005b) From realpolitik to dingpolitik or how to make things public. In B. Latour, P. Weibel and M. Zentrum für Kunst und (Eds) *Making things public: atmospheres of democracy.* Cambridge, MA; London: ZKM/Center for Art and Media in Karlsruhe: MIT Press. Pp. 14–44.

Latour, B. (2013) *An inquiry into modes of existence: an anthropology of the moderns.* Cambridge, MA: Harvard University Press.

Latour, B. and Woolgar, S. (1986) *Laboratory life: the construction of scientific facts.* Princeton, NJ: Princeton University Press.

Law, J. (1991) Strategies of power: power, discretion and strategy. In J. Law (Ed) *A sociology of monsters: essays on power, technology, and domination.* London; New York: Routledge. Pp. 165–192.

Law, J. (2004) *After method: mess in social science research.* London; New York: Routledge.

Law, J. (2007) Pinboards and books: juxtaposing, learning and materiality. In D. Kritt and L.T. Winegar (Eds) *Education and technology: critical perspectives, possible futures.* Lanham, MD: Lexington Books. Pp. 125–150.

Law, J. (2009) Actor network theory and material semiotics. In B. Turner (Ed) *The new Blackwell companion to social theory.* Oxford: Blackwell. Pp. 141–158.

Law, J. (2011) *Heterogeneous engineering and tinkering.* Available at: www.hetero geneities.net/publications/Law2011HeterogeneousEngineeringAndTinkering.pdf

Law, J. and Singleton, V. (2000) Performing technology's stories: on social constructivism, performance, and performativity. *Technology and Culture* 41(4): 765–775.

Law, J. and Urry, J. (2004) Enacting the social. *Economy & Society* 33(3): 390–410.

Laws, S. (1990) *Issues of blood: the politics of menstruation.* Basingstoke: Macmillian.

Lecercle, J-J. (2002) Deleuze and language. Basingstoke: Palgrave MacMillan.

Lewis, M. (2012) Addiction as self-medication. *Psychology Today.* Available at: https://www.psychologytoday.com/blog/addicted-brains/201208/addiction-self-medication

Lindsay, J. (2009) Young Australians and the staging of intoxication and self-control. *Journal of Youth Studies* 12(4): 371–384.

Literat, I. (2013) 'A Pencil for your thoughts': participatory drawing as a visual research method with children and youth. *International Journal of Qualitative Methods* 12: 84–98.

Lury, C. and Wakeford, N. (Eds) (2012) *Inventive methods: the happening of the social.* Abington, Oxon; New York: Routledge.

MacGregor, S. (2017) *The politics of drugs: perceptions, power and policies.* London: Palgrave Macmillan.

MacLure, M. (2013) Classification or wonder? Coding as an analytic practice in qualitative research'. In R. Coleman and J. Ringrose (Eds) *Deleuze and research methodologies.* Edinburgh: Edinburgh University Press. Pp.164–184.

Malbon, B. (1999) *Clubbing: dancing, ecstasy, vitality: clubbing cultures and experience.* London: Routledge.

Malins, P. (2004) Machinic assemblages: Deleuze, Guattari and an ethico-aesthetics of drug use. *Janus Head* 7(1): 84–104.

Malins, P. (2007) City folds: injecting drug use and urban space. In A. Hickey-Moody and P. Malins (Eds) *Deleuzian encounters: studies in contemporary social issues.* Basingstoke: Palgrave Macmillan.

Malins, P. (2009) *An ethico-aesthetics of injecting drug use: body, space, memory, capital* (PhD thesis). The University of Melbourne. Available at: https://minerva-access.unimelb.edu.au/handle/11343/35163

Malins, P. (2011) An ethico-aesthetics of heroin chic: art, cliche and capitalism. In L. Guillaume and J. Hughes (Eds) *Deleuze and the body.* Edinburgh: Edinburgh University Press. Pp. 165–188.

Malins, P. (2017) Desiring assemblages: a case for desire over pleasure in critical drug studies. *International Journal of Drug Policy* 49: 126–132.

Malins, P., Fitzgerald, J.L. and Threadgold, T. (2006) Spatial 'folds': the entwining of bodies, risks and city spaces for women injecting drug users in Melbourne's central business district. *Gender, Place and Culture* 13(5): 509–527.

Manning, P. (2007) *Drugs and popular culture: drugs, media and identity in contemporary society.* Uffculme: Willan Publishing.

Martin, A., Myers, N. and Viseu, A. (2015) The politics of care in technoscience. *Sociological Review* 45(5): 625–641.

Mason, J. (2010) *Creative interviewing* [Video file]. Available at: www.ncrm.ac.uk/resources/video/realities/creative.php

Massumi, B. (1998) Event horizon. In J. Brouwer (Ed) *The art of the accident.* Rotterdam: Dutch Architecture Institute. Pp. 154–168

Massumi, B. (2002) *Parables for the virtual: movement, affect, sensation.* Durham, NC: Duke University Press.

Massumi, B. (2015) *Politics of affect.* Cambridge: Polity Press.

McKeganey, N. (2012) Harm reduction at the crossroads and the rediscovery of drug user abstinence. *Drugs: Education, Prevention, and Policy* 19(4): 276–283.

McLean, K. (2011) The biopolitics of needle exchange in the United States. *Critical Public Health* 21(1): 71–79.

Measham, F. (2000) Locating leisure: feminist, historical and structural perspectives on young people's leisure, substance use and social divisions in 1990s British pubs and clubs (Unpublished PhD thesis). University of Manchester.

Measham, F. (2002) 'Doing gender' 'doing drugs': conceptualizing the gendering of drugs cultures. *Contemporary Drug Problems* 29(2): 335.

Measham, F. (2004) Play space: historical and socio-cultural reflections on drugs, licensed leisure locations, commercialisation and control. *International Journal of Drug Policy* 15(5–6): 337–345.

Measham, F. (2006) The new policy mix: alcohol, harm minimisation, and determined drunkenness in contemporary society. *International Journal of Drug Policy* 17(4): 258–268.

Measham, F. and Brain, K. (2005) 'Binge' drinking, British alcohol policy and the new culture of intoxication. *Crime, Media, Culture* 1(3): 262–263.

Measham, F. and Shiner, M. (2009) The legacy of 'normalisation': the role of classical and contemporary criminological theory in understanding young people's drug use. *International Journal of Drug Policy* 20(6): 502–508.

Meyer, M. (2008) On the boundaries and partial connections between amateurs and professionals. *Museum and Society* 6(1): 38–53.

Michael, M. and Rosengarten, M. (2012) Medicine: experimentation, politics, emergent bodies. *Body & Society* 18(3–4): 1–17.

Michael, M. and Rosengarten, M. (2013) *Innovation and biomedicine: ethics, evidence and expectation in HIV*. Basingstoke: Palgrave Macmillan.

Mol, A. (1999) Ontological politics. A word and some questions. *The Sociological Review* 47: 74–89.

Mol, A. (2002) *The body multiple: ontology in medical practice*. Durham, NC; London: Duke University Press.

Mol, A. (2008) *The logic of care: health and the problem of patient choice*. London; New York: Routledge.

Mol, A. (2010) Actor-network theory: sensitive terms and enduring tensions. *Kölner Zeitschrift für Soziologie und Sozialpsychologie* 50(1): 253–269.

Mol, A. (2014) *Physio-moral accounts: eating pleasures and destructions*. Paper presented at 'HARC dialogues: the value of eating'. Royal Holloway University of London, 13 March. Available at: http://backdoorbroadcasting.net/2014/03/annemarie-mol-physio-moral-accounts-eating-pleasures-and-destructions/

Mol, A. and Law, J. (2004) Embodied action, enacted bodies. The example of hypoglycaemia. *Body & Society* 10(2): 43–62.

Mol, A., Moser, I. and Pols, J. (Eds) (2010) *Care in practice: on tinkering in clinics, homes and farms*. Bielefeld; Piscataway, NJ: Transcript.

Monaghan, M. (2012) The recent evolution of UK drug strategies: from maintenance to behaviour change. *People, Place & Policy Online* 6(1): 29–40.

Moore, D. (2004) Governing street-based injecting drug users: a critique of heroin overdose prevention in Australia. *Social Science & Medicine* 59(7): 1547–1557.

Moore, D. and Fraser, S. (2006) Putting at risk what we know: reflecting on the drug-using subject in harm reduction and its political implications. *Social Science & Medicine* 62(12): 3035–3047.

Moreira, T. (2010) Now or later? Individual disease and care collectives in the memory clinic. In A. Mol, I. Moser and J. Pols (Eds) *Care in practice: on tinkering in clinics, homes and farms*. Bielefeld; Piscataway, NJ: Transcript. Pp. 119–141.

Mugford, S. (1993) Harm reduction: does it lead where its proponents imagine? In N. Heather, A. Wodak, E. Nadelmann and P. O'Hare (Eds) *Psychoactive drugs and harm reduction: from faith to science*. London: Whurr. Pp. 21–34.

Müller, M. (2015) Assemblages and actor-networks: rethinking socio-material power, politics and space. *Geography Compass* 9(1): 27–41.

Nature (2014, February 6) Editorial: animal farm. *Nature* 506: 5.

NDTMS (National Drug Treatment Monitoring System) (2016) Adult substance misuse statistics from the National Drug Treatment Monitoring System (NDTMS): 1st April 2015 to 31st March 2016. Available at: http://webarchive.nationalarchives.gov.uk/20170807160711/www.nta.nhs.uk/statistics.aspx

NDTMS (National Drug Treatment Monitoring System) (2017) Adult substance misuse statistics from the National Drug Treatment Monitoring System (NDTMS): 1 April 2016 to 31 March 2017. Available at: https://assets.publishing.service.gov.uk/government/uploads/system/uploads/attachment_data/file/658056/Adult-statistics-from-the-national-drug-treatment-monitoring-system-2016-2017.pdf

Nettleton, S., Neale, J. and Pickering, L. (2011) 'I don't think there's much of a rational mind in a drug addict when they are in the thick of it': towards an embodied analysis of recovering heroin users. *Sociology of Health & Illness* 33(3): 341–355.

Nettleton, S., Neale, J. and Pickering, L. (2013) 'I just want to be normal': an analysis of discourses of normality among recovering heroin users. *Health* 17(2): 174–190.

NHS (National Health Service, National Treatment Agency for Substance Misuse) (2012) *Medications in recovery: re-orientating drug dependence treatment*. Available at: www.nta.nhs.uk/uploads/medications-in-recovery-main-report3.pdf

NIDA (National Institute on Drug Abuse) (2015) National Institute on Drug Abuse [website]. Available at: www.drugabuse.gov/

Nutt, D. (2012, December 3) Drugs are taken for pleasure - realise this and we can start to reduce harm. *The Guardian*. Available at: www.theguardian.com/commentisfree/2012/dec/03/drugs-pleasure-reduce-harm

O'Hare, P.A., Newcombe, R., Mathews, A., Buning, E.C. and Drucker, E. (1992) *The reduction of drug-related harm*. London; New York: Routledge.

O'Malley, P. (2002) Drugs, risks and freedoms: illicit drug 'use' and 'misuse' under neo-liberal governance. In G. Hughes, E. McLaughlin and J. Muncie (Eds) *Crime prevention and community safety: new directions*. London; Thousand Oaks, CA; Delhi: Sage Publications. Pp. 279–296.

O'Malley, P. and Valverde, M. (2004) Pleasure, freedom and drugs: the uses of 'pleasure' in liberal governance of drug and alcohol consumption. *Sociology* 38(1): 25–42.

ONS (Office for National Statistics) (2015) *Deaths related to drug poisoning in England and Wales: 2014 registrations*. Available at: www.ons.gov.uk/people populationandcommunity/birthsdeathsandmarriages/deaths/bulletins/deathsrelatedtodrugpoisoninginenglandandwales/2015-09-03#main-points

ONS (Office for National Statistics) (2018) Deaths related to drug poisoning in England and Wales: 2017 registrations. Available at: https://www.ons.gov.uk/peoplepopulationandcommunity/birthsdeathsandmarriages/deaths/bulletins/deathsrelatedtodrugpoisoninginenglandandwales/2017registrations

Parker, H., Aldridge, J. and Measham, F. (1998) *Illegal leisure: the normalization of adolescent drug use*. London; New York: Routledge.

Parkin, S. G. (2013) *Habitus and drug using environments: health, place and lived-experience*. Farnham: Ashgate.

Phaphides, P. (1997, Jun 1) Rave new world. *Time Out*. Pp. 11–18.

PHE (Public Health England) (2017) Health matters: preventing drug misuse deaths. Available at: www.gov.uk/government/publications/health-matters-preventing-drug-misuse-deaths/health-matterspreventing-drug-misuse-deaths

Pienaar, K. and Dilkes-Frayne, E. (2017) Telling different stories, making new realities: the ontological politics of 'addiction' biographies. *International Journal of Drug Policy* 44: 145–154.

Pienaar, K., Fraser, S., Kokanovic, R., Moore, D., Treloar, C. and Dunlop, A. (2015) New narratives, new selves: complicating addiction in online alcohol and other drug resources. *Addiction Research & Theory* 23(6): 499–509.

Pienaar, K., Moore, D., Fraser, S., Kokanovic, R., Treloar, C. and Dilkes-Frayne, E. (2017) Diffracting addicting binaries: an analysis of personal accounts of alcohol and other drug 'addiction'. *International Journal of Drug Policy* 21(5): 519–537.

Pierides, D. and Woodman, D. (2012) Object-oriented sociology and organizing in the face of emergency: Bruno Latour, Graham Harman and the material turn. *The British Journal of Sociology* 63(4): 662–679.

Pink, S. (2009) *Doing sensory ethnography*. Los Angeles, CA; London; New Delhi; Singapore; Washington, DC: SAGE Publications.

Poulsen, M. (2015) Embodied subjectivities: bodily subjectivity and changing boundaries in post-human alcohol practices. *Contemporary Drug Problems* 42(1): 3–19.

Povinelli, E.A. (2018) Holding up the world, part II: time/bank, effort/embankments. *E-flux* 58. Available at: www.e-flux.com/journal/58/61147/holding-up-the-world-part-ii-time-bank-effort-embankments/

Preda, A. (1999) The turn to things: arguments for a sociological theory of things. *Sociological Quarterly* 40: 347–366.

Puig de la Bellacasa, M. (2017) *Matters of care: speculative ethics in more than human worlds.* Minneapolis: University of Minnesota Press.

Race, K. (2008) The use of pleasure in harm reduction: perspectives from the history of sexuality. *International Journal of Drug Policy* 19(5): 417–423.

Race, K. (2009) *Pleasure consuming medicine: the queer politics of drugs.* Durham; London: Duke University Press.

Race, K. (2014) Complex events: drug effects and emergent causality. *Contemporary Drug Problems* 41(3): 301–334.

Race, K. (2017) Thinking with pleasure: experimenting with drugs and drug research. *International Journal of Drug Policy* 49: 144–149.

Race, K. (2018) *The gay science: intimate experiments with the problem of HIV.* Abingdon, Oxon; New York: Routledge.

Rajchman, J. (2000) *The Deleuze connections.* Cambridge, MA; London: The MIT Press.

Reinarman, C. and Levine, H.G. (Eds) (1997) *Crack in America: demon drugs and social justice.* Berkeley: University of California Press.

Restivo, S. (2005) Politics of Latour. *Organization & Environment* 8(1): 111–115.

Restivo, S. (2011) *Red, black, and objective.* Aldershot: Ashgate.

Reynold, S. (1999) *Generation ecstasy: into the world of techno and rave culture.* New York: Routledge.

Rhodes, T. (1995) Theorising and researching 'risk': notes on the social relations of risk in heroin users' lifestyles. In P. Aggleton, P. Hart and P. Davies (Eds) *AIDS: sexuality, safety and risk.* London: Taylor and Francis. Pp. 125–144.

Rhodes, T. (1997) Risk theory in epidemic times: sex, drugs and the social organisation of 'risk behaviour'. *Sociology of Health & Illness* 19(2): 208–227.

Rhodes, T. (2002) The 'risk environment': a framework for understanding and reducing drug-related harm. *International Journal of Drug Policy* 13(2): 85–94.

Rhodes, T. (2009) Risk environments and drug harms: a social science for harm reduction approach. *International Journal of Drug Policy* 20(3): 193–201.

Rhodes, T. (2018) The becoming of methadone in Kenya: how an intervention's implementation constitutes recovery potential. *Social Science & Medicine* 201: 71–79.

Rhodes, T. and Hartnoll, R. (1996) *AIDS, drugs and prevention: perspectives on individual and community action.* London: Routledge.

Rhodes, T., Closson, R., Guise, A. Paparini, S. and Strathdee, S. (2016) Towards 'evidence-making intervention' approaches in the social science of implementation science: the making of methadone in East Africa. *International Journal of Drug Policy* 30: 17–26.

Rhodes, T., Mikhailova, L., Sarang, A., Lowndes, C., Rylkov, A., Khutorskoy, M., et al. (2003) Situational factors associated with drug injecting, risk reduction and syringe exchange practices in Togliatti city, Russian Federation: a qualitative study of micro risk environment. *Social Science and Medicine* 57: 39–54.

Rhodes, T., Rance, J., Fraser, S. and Treloar, C. (2017) The intimate relationship as a site of social protection: partnerships between people who inject drugs. *Social Science & Medicine* 180: 125–134.

Rhodes, T., Singer, M., Bourgois, P., Friedman, S.R. and Strathdee, S.A. (2005) The social structural production of HIV risk among injecting drug users. *Social Science & Medicine* 61: 1026–1044.

Rhodes, T., Wagner, K., Strathdee, S.A., Shannon, K., Davidson, P. and Bourgois, P. (2012) Structural violence and structural vulnerability within the risk environment: theoretical and methodological perspectives for a social epidemiology of HIV risk among injection drug users and sex workers. In P. O'Campo and J.R. Dunn (Eds) *Rethinking social epidemiology*. New York: Springer. Pp. 205–223.

Rinella, M.A. (2010) *Pharmakon: Plato, drug culture, and identity in ancient Athens*. Lanham, MD: Lexington Books.

Ringrose, J. and Coleman, R. Looking and desiring machines: a feminist Deleuzian mapping of bodies and affects. In R. Coleman and J. Ringrose (Eds) *Deleuze and research methodologies*. Edinburgh: Edinburgh University Press. Pp. 125–145.

Robinson, T.E. and Berridge, K.C. (2003) Addiction. *Annual Review of Psychology* 54: 25–53.

Roe, G. (2005) Harm reduction as paradigm: is better than bad good enough? The origins of harm reduction. *Critical Public Health* 15(3): 243–250.

Rose, M. and Wylie, J. (2006) Animating landscape. *Environment and Planning D: Society and Space* 24: 475–479.

Rose, N. (2000) Government and control. *British Journal of Criminology* 40: 321–339.

Rose, N., O'Malley, P. and Valverde, M. (2006) Governmentality. *Annual Review of Law and Social Science* 2: 83–104.

Rosengarten, M. and Michael, M. (2009) Rethinking the bioethical enactment of medically drugged bodies: paradoxes of using anti-HIV drug therapy as a technology for prevention. *Science as Culture* 18(2): 183–199.

Rudy, A.P. and Gareau, B.J. (2005) Actor-network theory, Marxist economics, and Marxist political ecology. *Capitalism Nature Socialism* 16(4): 85–90.

Sarang, A., Rhodes, T., Sheon, N. and Page, K. (2010) Policing drug users in Russia: risk, fear, and structural violence. *Substance Use & Misuse* 45(6): 813–864.

Savransky, M. (2016) Thinking bodies [unpublished conference paper]. Biopolitics and psychosomatics: participating bodies (8 Jul). University of Cambridge.

Savransky, M., Wilkie, A. and Rosengarten, M. (2017) The lure of possible futures: on speculative research. In A. Wilkie, M. Savransky and M. Rosengarten (Eds) *Speculative research: the lure of possible futures*. Abingdon, Oxon; New York: Routledge. Pp. 1–18.

Schwarz, O. (2013) Bending forward, one step backward: on the sociology of tasting techniques. *Cultural Sociology* 7(4): 415–430.

Sedgwick, E.K. (1993) Epidemics of the will. In E.K. Sedgwick (Ed). *Tendencies*. Durham: Duke University Press. Pp. 130–143.

Seear, K. and Moore, D. (2014) Complexity: researching alcohol and other drugs in a multiple world. *Contemporary Drug Problems* 41(3): 295–300.

Seear, K., Fraser, S. and Lenton, E. (2010) Guilty or angry? The politics of emotion in accounts of hepatitis C transmission. *Contemporary Drug Problems* 37: 619–638.

Semetsky, I. (2011) Becoming-other: developing the ethics of integration. *Policy Futures in Education* 9(1): 138–144.

Shilling, C. (2008) *Changing bodies: habit, crisis and creativity.* London: Sage.

Shilling, C. (2012) *The body and social theory* (3rd ed.). London: Sage.

Singhal, A. and Rattine-Flaherty, E. (2006) Pencils and photos as tools of communicative research and praxis: analyzing Minga Perú's quest for social justice in the Amazon. *International Communication Gazette* 68(4): 313–330.

SMART recovery (n.d.) About SMART recovery. Available at: www.smartrecovery. org.uk/about-the-smart-recovery-programme/

Somatosphere (2014) *A reader's guide to the 'ontological turn'.* Available at: http:// somatosphere.net/series/ontology-2

SSDP (Students for Sensible Drug Policy UK) (2014) *An open letter to Russell Brand...* Available at: www.ssdp.org.uk/an-open-letter-to-russell-brand/

Stagoll, C. (2010) Event. In A. Parr (Ed) *The Deleuze dictionary.* Edinburgh: Edinburgh University Press. Pp. 89–91.

Stengers, I. (1997) *Power and invention: situating science.* Minneapolis: University of Minnesota Press.

Stewart, K. (2007) *Ordinary affects.* Durham; London: Duke University Press.

Stewart, K. (2011) Atmospheric attunements. *Environment and Planning D: Society and Space* 29: 445–453.

Stimson, G. (2000) Blair declares war: the unhealthy state of British drug policy. *International Journal of Drug Policy* 11(4): 259–264.

Stimson G (2007) 'Harm reduction-coming of age': a local movement with global impact. *International Journal of Drug Policy* 18: 67–69.

Strathern, M. (1991) *Partial connections.* Savage, MD: Rowman & Littlefield Publishers.

Szmigin, I.T., Griffin, C., Hackley, C., Bengry-Howell, A. and Mistral, W. (2008) Re-framing 'binge drinking' as calculated hedonism: empirical evidence from the UK. *International Journal of Drug Policy* 19(5): 359–366.

Tarr, J., Cornish, F., Gonzalez-Polledo, E. and Bicquelet, A. (2014) *Communicating chronic pain.* Milton Keynes: Lightning Source.

Thomas, H. and Ahmed, J. (Eds) (2004) *Cultural bodies: ethnography and theory.* Malden, MA: Blackwell Pub.

Thrift, N. (2000) Still life in nearly present time: the object of nature. *Body & Society* 6(3–4): 34–57.

Tronto, J. (1993) *Moral boundaries: a political argument for an ethic of care.* New York: Routledge.

valentine, k. (2007) Methadone maintenance treatment and making up people. *Sociology* 41(3): 497–514.

Valverde, M. (1998) *Diseases of the will: alcohol and the dilemmas of freedom.* Cambridge: Cambridge University Press.

Van Schipstal, I., Mishra, S., Berning, M. and Murray, H. (2016) Harm reduction from below: on sharing and caring in drug use. *Contemporary Drug Problems* 43(3): 199–215.

Vargas, E.V. (2010) Tarde on drugs, or measure against suicide. In M. Candea (Ed) *The social after Gabriel Tarde: debates and assessments.* London: Routledge. Pp. 208–230.

Vitellone, N. (2003a) The syringe as a prosthetic. *Body & Society* 9(3): 37–52.

Vitellone, N. (2003b) The rush: needle fixation or technical materialization? *Journal for Cultural Research* 7(2): 165–177.

Vitellone, N. (2004) Habitus and social suffering: culture, addiction and the syringe. In L. Adkins and B. Skeggs (Eds) *Feminism after Bourdieu*. Oxford: Blackwell Publishing/The Sociological Review. Pp. 129–148.

Vitellone, N. (2010) Just another night in the shooting gallery? The syringe, space, and affect. *Environment and Planning D: Society and Space* 28: 867–880.

Vitellone, N. (2015) Syringe sociology. *The British Journal of Sociology* 66: 373–390.

Vitellone, N. (2017) *Science of the syringe*. London: Routledge.

Vrecko, S. (2010) Birth of a brain disease: science, the state and addiction neuropolitics. *History of the Human Sciences* 23(4): 52–67.

Walkerdine, V. (2010) Communal beingness and affect: an exploration of trauma in an ex-industrial community. *Body & Society* 16(1): 91–116.

Warburton, D. (1994) *Pleasure: the politics and the reality*. New York: John Wiley and Sons.

Weinberg, D. (2002) On the embodiment of addiction. *Body & Society* 8(4): 1–19.

Weinberg, D. (2013) Post-humanism, addiction and the loss of self-control: reflections on the missing core in addiction science. *International Journal of Drug Policy* 24(3): 173–181.

Whatmore, S. (2006) Materialist returns: practising cultural geography in and for a more-than-human world. *Cultural Geographies* 13(4): 600–609.

Whatmore, S. (2013) Earthly powers: thinking through flooding. *Theory, Culture & Society* 30(7–8): 33–50.

Wilkie, A., Savransky, M. and Rosengarten, M. (Eds) (2017) *Speculative research: the lure of possible futures*. Abingdon, Oxon; New York: Routledge.

Wilson, A. (2007) *Northern soul: music, drugs and subcultural identity*. Cullompton: Willan.

Wintour, P. (2015, Jul 29). Obese people and drug users who refuse treatment could have benefits cut. *The Guardian*. Available at: www.theguardian.com/society/2015 /jul /29/benefits-drugs-alcohol-obesity-refusing-treatment-review

Witteveen, E., Van Ameijden, E.J.C. and Schippers, G.M. (2006) Motives for and against injecting drug use among young adults in Amsterdam: qualitative findings and considerations for disease prevention. *Substance Use & Misuse* 41(6–7): 1001–1016.

Wollaston, S. (2017, Oct 8) Louis Theroux: dark states – heroin town review: bleak as hell. *The Guardian*. Available at: www.theguardian.com/tv-and-radio/2017/ oct/08/louis-theroux-dark-states-heroin-town-review-bleak-as-hell

Woods, N. (2016) Better parked than dead. *Volteface*. Available at: http://volteface. me/features/heroin-and-healing/?utm_source=twitter&utm_medium=social& utm_campaign=SocialWarfare

Woolgar, S., Cheniti, T. Lezaun, J., Neyland, D., Sugden, C. and Toennesen, C. (no date) *A turn to ontology in STS?* Available at: www.sbs.ox.ac.uk/sites/default/ files/Research_Areas/Science_And_Technology/Docs/JohnLaw.pdf

Young, J. (1971) *The drugtakers: the social meaning of drug use*. London: MacGibbon & Kee.

Zinberg, N.E. (1984) *Drug, set, and setting: the basis for controlled intoxicant use*. New Haven, CT: Yale University Press.

Index

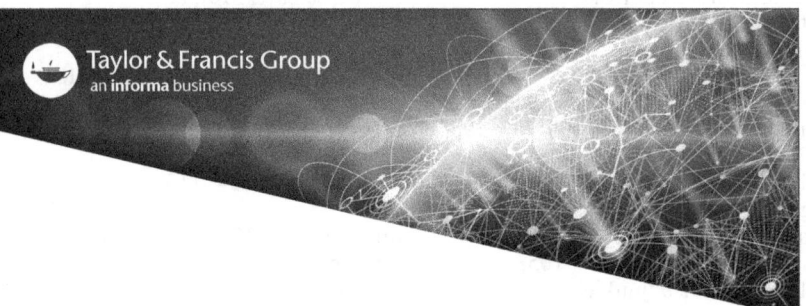
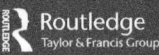
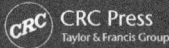